To Your Health!

To Your Health!

*Two Physicians
Explore the
Health Benefits
of Wine*

David N. Whitten, M.D., Ph.D.,
and Martin R. Lipp, M.D.

HarperCollinsWest
An Imprint of HarperCollins*Publishers*

HarperCollins®, ■ ®, and HarperCollinsWest™ are trademarks of HarperCollins Publishers Inc.

Book design by Ralph Fowler
Set in Trump Mediäval

FIRST HARPERCOLLINSWEST PAPERBACK EDITION
PUBLISHED IN 1996

Library of Congress Cataloging-in-Publication Data

Whitten, David N.
  To your health : two physicians explore the
health benefits of wine / David N. Whitten and
Martin R. Lipp.—
1st ed.
  p. cm.
  Includes bibliographical references and index.
  ISBN 0–06–258514–2 (cloth)
  ISBN 0–06–258599–1 (pbk.)
  1. Wine—Health aspects. I. Lipp, Martin R.
  II. Title.
RA784.L56 1994   93–5437
613'.3—dc20   CIP

96 97 98 99 00 ❖ RRD(H) 10 9 8 7 6 5 4 3 2 1

For

Karen, Laura, Emily, Sarah, and David

and for

Natividad, Michelle, and Melissa

Contents

A CAUTION TO THE READER

Very little information on the topic of alcohol and health remains free from subjective bias. We, the authors, have done our best to base our conclusions on medical facts as we understand them. Still, the judgments and recommendations in the pages ahead represent our opinions. Before applying these opinions to your own personal health decisions, please discuss them with your physician and others whose objectivity and common sense you value.

Introduction

When patients ask us about the risks and benefits of drinking wine, we like to answer with a story about scientific research. Two lab rats are sitting in their cage as a couple of researchers enter the room. The older, more experienced rat says to the younger one, "Stay away from scientists." "Why?" asks the younger. "They cause cancer," replies the other.

As with most black humor, there is something to be learned from this story. First, it is true that practically any substance imaginable will cause biological mischief if crammed into laboratory animals in sufficient quantities. Second, whether consciously or not, scientists habitually create and report such biological mischief because it often leads to more research grants, promotion, and occasional notoriety, as well as scientific knowledge. If selected fragments from those reports will sell newspapers or fit the political view of some special interest group who can use them to support their own agenda, the fragments will become "news."

Thus, the "health scare of the week" has become a fixture in our lives. Recently, we have seen reports that cancer comes from preservatives in hot dogs, herbicides on fruit, drugs in cows' milk, and alcohol in wine. Such reports generate an interesting series of counter-reports, resulting in a growing list of cancer-thwarting foods: green tea, garlic, onions, broccoli, and, yes, wine, among others.

Of course, health claims for foods are not new: Ancient civilizations used such items as oranges as antidotes for various poisons, as a treatment for tapeworm, and as a specific medication for the fevers caused by the plague. One hundred years ago, the medical literature regarded wine as a restorative, a stimulant, and a choice analgesic for many of the body's aches.

What *has* changed, however, is our recent ability to make more accurate analyses of those same claims. We can now analyze various foods for their active ingredients, quantify chemical components at incredibly minute concentrations, monitor biological processes at a cellular and subcellular level, conduct enormous epidemiological stud-

INTRODUCTION

ies, and, thanks to computers, process vast amounts of statistical data in a matter of seconds.

On the other hand, our latter-twentieth-century ability to communicate instantly with one another over the entire globe explodes some very shaky conjecture. Via the expedient of press releases, we are offered "the latest scientific information." Yet merely reporting a news item as fact does not make it so, and in order to gain scientific objectivity we are more dependent than ever on discerning and responsible news gathering.

Unfortunately, hard facts linking individual food items with either specific health risks or benefits are in exceedingly short supply. It comes as no surprise then that reputable medical observers are quick to acknowledge an enormous gap between public concern and actual scientific knowledge.

When it comes to wine and health, each month seems to yield a plethora of highly publicized claims, many seemingly contradicting what was reported only a few months before: "Wine can give you lead poisoning." "Red wine lowers your cholesterol." "Wine raises your blood pressure." "Wine helps prevent heart attacks." "Wine clears the thinking of Alzheimer's patients." "Sulfites in wine kill asthma sufferers." "A pregnant woman who drinks wine condemns her child to an impaired life." And so on, and so on.

What should the public do with such information? Is it all nonsense or just some of it, and how can one tell the difference? What should be the practical impact of such information? How should the reasonably health-conscious citizen change dietary habits, if at all? Because we live in a culture whose views on alcoholic beverages tend to be dominated by abusers, on the one hand, and neoprohibitionists, on the other, these questions are far more confusing with regard to wine than with other foodstuffs. Today, 70 percent of Americans drink alcoholic beverages while 30 percent do not; few individuals in either group regard spokespeople in the other as being dispassionate on the subject.

The literature on this topic suffers a similar fate. If you begin reading about wine and health, you quickly discover that much of the printed material comes from people with axes to grind. We are talking about multibillion-dollar industries here—and not just the wine industry.

We all know that we must be wary of a salesperson's claims, but many in the general public do not fully appreciate that antialcohol forces also sell something. This group now represents a huge industry—in the billions of dollars—with thousands of jobs to preserve and budgets and empires to protect and expand. This group includes not only religious teetotalers and neoprohibitionists, but also many tens of thousands of recovery and alcoholism treatment people whose livelihoods require the constant stoking of public anxiety about alcohol in any of its forms.

Of course, it is far easier to scare people than to reassure them. To scare, one has only to raise doubt; to reassure generally requires replacing doubt with certainty—and certainty can be a fragile commodity. This is especially true when much of what we know remains tentative and requires sorting the truth and the facts from conflicting studies.

Another problem in maintaining objectivity arises from the source of the information itself. Scientific knowledge does not grow in a vacuum: It springs from soil fertilized by historical tradition, cultural values, and especially political pressures and the influence generated by those who fund research. For example, the National Institute of Alcohol Abuse and Alcoholism (the NIAAA—whose name describes its concerns) controls almost 80 percent of alcohol-related research in the United States. Thus, research focuses on alcohol-related problems rather than alcohol-related benefits. For example, the overwhelming bulk of our knowledge of alcohol's biological effects derives from studies of alcholics and others who regularly drink to excess. High-quality studies on the effects of light, regular drinking barely exist in the federally sponsored arena.

If we here are to avoid similar pitfalls as authors, we must first define our terms as well as our own biases.

First, the term *moderate drinking* means many things to different people, and the definitions tend to be culturally dependent. To some American authorities, moderate drinking means a maximum of four drinks a week, whereas to the British, it means up to five drinks per day. For our purposes, we will concentrate on wine drinking at the level of one or two four-ounce glasses of table wine per day, and we will call this amount "light, regular wine consumption."

We have chosen this amount primarily because most scientific papers that relate health to nonabusive alcohol consumption use the same figures, and because, practically speaking, no one can order less than this amount in a restaurant or social setting. Moreover, under ordinary circumstances, for a 130-pound woman, one glass of wine will produce a blood alcohol concentration (BAC) equivalent to that of two glasses for a 180-pound man, and for either individual these amounts will produce a BAC well under 0.08 percent, the most stringent threshold for drunken driving currently legislated in the United States: 0.08 milligrams alcohol per 100 cubic centimeters blood. The BAC would be even lower when food accompanies the wine, as is usually the case.

It is important to note that "regular" means *daily* consumption. We emphasize this fact because we do not wish to mislead readers into believing that drinking seven to fourteen glasses only once a week on Saturdays averages out to the same total consumption as one or two glasses each day.

Thus, for the sake of this book, "light, regular wine consumption" means either one daily mealtime glass of table wine for a 130-pound woman or two daily mealtime glasses for a 180-pound man.

It makes sense at this point to report our own background and biases, and we have several. First, we are physicians specializing in emergency medicine. Our combined experience totals almost forty years in busy metropolitan emergency medicine departments. We cannot discuss any alcoholic beverage without an awareness of its potential for abuse. We have seen too many victims of motor vehicle accidents, too many victims of violence, to neglect this side of the equation. Trying to patch up smelly, abusive, spitting, vomiting, swearing, uncooperative drunks who have just driven their vehicle into a carload of innocent victims creates a loathing hard to comprehend unless you have shared the experience.

Obviously, this background forces us to acknowledge the problem of alcohol abuse from the outset. In fact, the greatest health risk associated with light, regular wine consumption may be the small but definite potential for it to escalate into alcohol abuse, and we will discuss this very risk in the pages ahead. Still, light, regular wine consumption, by definition, differs from abuse and, as we shall see, involves qualitatively different benefits and hazards.

Second, we both have strong groundings in the sciences. In addition to our medical degrees, one of us earned a Ph.D. in physiology, and we both have published independent research, adding our bit to the cumulative storehouse of scientific information. Thus we believe in the value of objectivity. We believe in careful, thorough research, and we value balanced and careful analysis. We see science as a tool, a method, and a way of thinking that has great value. We also know that what sometimes masquerades as science often has little to do with common sense. Our own credentials free us from overawe at the credentials of others, and we know that credentials alone can never adequately substitute for scientific rigor. Therefore, we approach scientific reports, whether they support our biases or not, with a certain degree of skepticism.

Third, we are concerned citizens, and we feel a strong vested interest in sensible public policy—especially in medical and health arenas—based on solid reality, rather than rumors, emotions, and the political pressures of prevailing special interest groups. Certainly enough real dangers exist in the world that the government need not waste its time or finite resources scaring the public about dangers that have little or no statistical basis in fact.

Fourth, we are both regular, light-to-moderate wine drinkers. One of us grew up in a family of teetotalers, the other in a family where wine was consumed primarily as part of religious rituals. Now, both of us drink wine with meals and in social situations, with friends and family. Though we currently see our wine consumption as part of a healthy lifestyle, we believe ourselves willing to change if compelling medical evidence to the contrary exists now or were to come to light in the future. Just such evidence led one of us to cease pipe smoking and to refrain from motorcycle riding. The benefits and pleasures simply did not compensate for the risk involved.

Finally, we are both parents, one with four children and one with two. To the extent that we can, we want to protect our children from danger. We are concerned about teaching our children how to drink responsibly. Because 70 percent of our nation's adults do drink, chances are our kids will at least try alcoholic beverages at some point in their lives. How can we teach them to drink sensibly and with moderation when they are taught at school and elsewhere that alcohol is the most abused drug in the world, that use equals abuse? If they see their parents drinking wine with meals most nights and label the experience as "a form of drug abuse," as taught by some of their teachers, does that make them more or less able to cope with the genuine dangers of street drug abuse? How can we discuss the importance of responsible drinking with them when agencies like the NIAAA refuse even to use the term *responsible alcohol use*, on the grounds that all use involves some risk? As physicians and parents, we know that everything of value in life—from love and marriage, to the practice of medicine, to a walk on the seashore, to foodstuffs as common as fish, fruit, and milk—all involve some risk. How can we teach our children to see risk as a continuum rather than an all-or-nothing phenomenon, to help them assess risk thoughtfully and realistically as it applies to their own lives, to balance risk and reward, and then help them make sensible decisions? How do we teach them about age-appropriate behavior?

The challenges inherent in these questions led us to review the vast storehouse of information concerning wine and health. We sought to provide a sensible, balanced distillation of the available literature and to report it to you, the reader, in a fashion that will serve as a practical guide to determining whether light, regular wine drinking will help or hinder *your* health.

In seeking to make this determination, we applied four standards to the hundreds of research reports we examined. The first is as simple and commonsensical as it is rare in discussions on this topic: "compared to what?" Anyone can say that wine (or anything else, for that matter) helps you or harms you, but the assertion demands a standard of comparison. Because wine is a beverage, and usually people who decline to drink wine will choose to drink something else, we compare its health implications with similar standard servings of other common beverages, such as orange juice, whole milk, coffee, cola, and tap water. From time to time, as circumstances demand, we will compare wine to other foods as well, or to risks and benefits associated with such activities as recreational athletics.

The second standard concerns the quality of available research. What do we think we know, and how do we know it? What kind of research exists? Are the studies well designed? Have the data been subject to rigorous statistical analysis? Have the data been interpreted in a reasonable fashion, or do the interpretations themselves seem biased in any obvious manner?

Additionally, we will continuously ask, How many people should concern themselves with the results of this study, and to what degree? The implications differ if wine consumption alters the natural progression of a disease that kills hundreds of thousands each year, as opposed to a disease that involves only a handful of people over the course of decades.

Finally, we intend to apply the reasonable person test: Given that light, regular wine consumption appears to have a variety of effects depending on a number of different conditions; given that other beverages, foodstuffs, and activities have their own effects; and given that the quality of evidence varies enormously from excellent to slipshod—given all this, with as many specifics as we can provide—how should a reasonable person *respond*? In what way should all this information alter our behavior, if at all?

How one responds to the challenges posed by these questions is an intensely personal decision. Reasonable people will answer it differently, depending on how they weigh various personal values. However these challenges are met, we hope readers will be clear about our intent: We emphasize medical values in this book; medical and scientific literature remain our touchstones throughout. We have not considered such elusive matters as gastronomic preference, tradition, camaraderie, religious values, or even simple pleasure and enjoyment.

For better or worse, this book retains all the biases inherent in the medical model. Because the basis of medicine is pathology, this book necessarily emphasizes disease over well-being and the search for defects rather than for positive attributes. (The computerized directory of published articles in all the world's medical journals includes subcategories under "wine," for "toxicity" and "adverse effects" but no subcategories for "benefits" or "positive attributes.")

Finally, we intend that this book provide a sensible basis for making practical medical decisions about everyday behavior, free from exaggerated and sensational claims by special interest groups on either side of the contemporary debate. If we have succeeded in our goal—however limited that may be—then the enormous investment of time, effort, and thought devoted to this book will be well worthwhile.

In the pages ahead we will try to give the best, most reasoned answer possible, especially as wine affects our major health concerns.

Chapter 1

Wine and Nutrition

For centuries people have debated the relative health benefits of wine. It has been both praised as an aid to digestion
and reviled as a great evil. Today, it is sometimes called by
its supporters a "natural fruit beverage," an appetite stimulant, and even a food itself, whereas detractors view wine as
nothing but empty calories, an unnatural, toxic, and nutritionally unnecessary beverage.

To determine how much of each of these claims is true
and just what role wine should play in your daily diet, let's
look first at the nutritional standards we use to judge our
diets.

NUTRITIONAL STANDARDS

Though our interest in food—from taste to health effects—goes back as far as recorded history, nutrition as a science is in its infancy. Only in the past few decades have we had much in the way of genuinely scientific data concerning nutritional requirements, how various foods and food groups satisfy those requirements, and in what amounts. Moreover, the science of nutrition continues to evolve, so that much of what we think we know now will inevitably change with time.

Of course, every generation believes firmly the wisdom of its own era. Yet we do not need to look back very far to see how fragile that wisdom can be. In the early part of this century, the U.S. government recognized five food groups: vegetables and fruits, protein foods, cereals, sweets, and fats. Officials recommended that individuals consume almost a pound of sugar and nearly two ounces of fats such as lard, bacon, and butter per week! By the 1940s, the government recognized eight food groups for daily consumption (eggs occupied their own category, equal in value to each of the others). The four food groups most of us are familiar with were eventually devised in the 1960s. In addition to reorganizing these categories, officials then began to urge us to eat something from each group every day: meat, poultry, and fish; grains; dairy products; and fruits and vegetables. It was not until 1977 that the federal government recommended that we *limit* our intake of any dietary ingredient.

TO YOUR HEALTH!

Prior to that, the government suggested only that we *include* items from each food group in our diet.

Finally, in 1992, the Department of Agriculture graphically reorganized its recommendations from what had been more or less an equal-category "food wheel" into a new "food pyramid," providing different consumption levels for each category. The base is composed of grain products such as bread, cereal, rice, or pasta (6–11 servings recommended per day). Vegetables (3–5 servings) and fruits (2–4 servings) are next in importance. These are followed by milk, yogurt, or cheese (2–3 servings) and meat, fish, poultry, dried beans, eggs, or nuts (2–3 servings). The peak of the pyramid is composed of fats, oils, and sweets, and it is recommended that these be used sparingly. However, so much controversy erupted after the pyramid was introduced that it was withdrawn by May of the same year.

Americans clearly eat far more of many foods than experts consider advisable. According to the Surgeon General, women should cut their protein consumption by a third and men by almost 40 percent. Likewise, we consume two to four times more sodium than the National Research Council recommends. However, the single most important diet-related problem in the United States is obesity. According to the American Heart Association and the American Cancer Society, we consume about 25 percent more calories from fat than is healthy. Depending on how one defines the term, obesity afflicts probably 34 million adults; rates are higher among poor people and minorities. Generally, government reports estimate that a quarter of adults are sufficiently overweight to increase their risk for cardiovascular disease, diabetes, digestive diseases, cancer, and premature mortality.*

Recommended Daily Allowances

In order to help us determine what is a nutritious diet, the Food and Nutrition Board (FNB) of the National Academy of Sciences has published a list of Recommended Daily Allowances (the familiar "RDAs") since the early 1940s. Technically, RDAs are defined as the intake levels of "essential nutrients which, on the basis of scientific knowledge, are judged by the FNB to be adequate to meet the known nutrient needs of practically all healthy persons." This means that they should not be considered either acceptable minimums or permissible maximums but "target" figures that represent the center of an acceptable range. In other words, they are safe and adequate levels consumed as part of a normal diet.

*The reason for this excess is likely a result of cultural habit: Until the 1940s and 1950s, our country's primary nutritional concerns involved deficiency diseases such as rickets (vitamin D deficiency), pellagra (niacin), scurvy (vitamin C), and beriberi (thiamine). Though some cases of nutritional deficiency still exist in this country, they primarily involve "special" populations rather than the country as a whole. Iron deficiency, a condition common in 6–10 percent of young children and menstruating women, is one familiar example. Calcium deficiency may be a problem for some women, though a continuing series of controversies obscures the details. For the most part, nutritional deficiencies in this country remain a function of poverty, and, for the general population, experts worry more about diseases related to dietary excess and imbalance.

Like most figures produced by committee, RDAs are arrived at through argument, negotiation, and compromise. Specific recommendations vary with age, sex, and certain special conditions such as pregnancy and breast-feeding, and scientists on the FNB do not agree on recommendations for all nutrients. They have been able to develop RDAs for protein, some vitamins, and seven minerals, but nutrients conspicuously lacking on the RDA list include water, fiber, salt, carbohydrate, alcohol, and fat. Despite these caveats, RDAs represent the most widely acceptable figures available (Table A contains RDAs for both men and women ages twenty-five to fifty).

WINE, ALCOHOL, AND NUTRITION

Before we can determine how wine fares in terms of RDAs or any other measure of nutrition, we need to know what goes into making it. As most of us are aware, standard table wine comes from fermented grape juice. For the most part, the wine maker does little to speed or alter the "natural" fermentation process, in which yeasts turn most of the grape sugars into alcohol. Usually, the fermented juice is then clarified, sometimes using various additives or filters, aged for varying lengths of time, and then bottled. Despite these variables and a wide range of growing conditions, table wine tends to fit a fairly standard nutritional profile: It consists overwhelmingly of water with roughly 10 to 13

TABLE A
Recommended Daily Allowances for Men and Women

NUTRIENT	UNITS	MEN	WOMEN
Protein	grams	63	50
Vitamin A	micrograms	1000	800
Vitamin D	micrograms	5	5
Vitamin E	milligrams	10	8
Vitamin K	micrograms	80	65
Vitamin C	milligrams	60	60
Thiamine	milligrams	1.5	1.1
Riboflavin	milligrams	1.7	1.3
Niacin	milligrams	19	15
B-6	milligrams	2	1.6
Folacin	micrograms	200	180
B-12	micrograms	2	2
Calcium	milligrams	800	800
Phosphorus	milligrams	800	800
Magnesium	milligrams	350	280
Iron	milligrams	10	15
Zinc	milligrams	15	12

The FNB assumes that men weigh about 174 pounds and stand 5 feet 10 inches tall and women weigh 136 pounds and stand 5 feet 4 inches tall.

Adapted with permission from *Recommended Dietary Allowances: Tenth Edition.* Copyright © 1989 by the National Academy of Sciences. Courtesy of the National Academy Press, Washington, D.C.

TO YOUR HEALTH!

percent alcohol,* small amounts of carbohydrates, protein, and minerals, and trace amounts of vitamins.

Although there is a great deal of controversy concerning the social consequences of its use and abuse, alcohol is a relatively simple molecule, and at light, regular consumption levels scientists have no doubt concerning its primary contribution to human nutrition: It provides energy, which we customarily measure in calories. The secondary effects, all perceived with varying degrees of controversy, involve alcohol's impact on the body's need for and use of carbohydrates, fats, iron, vitamins, and the like.

Nutritional? Compared to What?

How then does wine compare with other foods, especially other beverages, in providing nutritional value for its caloric punch?

Table B provides a comparison of wine's nutritional content with that of other common beverages. If evaluated solely in terms of the "empty calories" charge, wine fares poorly vis-à-vis orange juice (at roughly the same number of calories) but well compared with cola. Coffee has almost no nutritional value but also lacks calories. Milk has more nutritional value but twice the calories per serving, with an added load of fat and cholesterol.

*Although alcoholic beverages are sometimes rated in terms of "proof" for commercial purposes, we will speak here only of percentages. Proof is a system based on two hundred units; therefore, "80 proof," the standard level of alcohol for hard liquor, is equivalent to 40-percent alcohol. Wine is generally 20 to 25 proof or 10–13 percent alcohol by volume.

TABLE B
Nutrient Content of Common Beverages:
Two Standard Servings

NUTRIENT	O. J.	COLA	COFFEE	WINE	MILK
Calories	222	310	8	164	300
Fat (g)	1	0	0	0	16
Carbohydrate (g)	51.6	80	1.6	3.2	22
Protein (g)	3.4	0	0.2	0.4	16
Vitamin A (IU)	992	0	0	0	0
Vitamin C (mg)	248	0	0	0	10
Thiamine (mg)	.44	0	0	0	0.2
Riboflavin (mg)	.14	0	0	.04	.84
Niacin (mg)	0.2	0	0.8	0.2	0.4
B-6 (mg)	.02	0	0	.06	.04
Folacin (mcg)	0	0	0	2.3	74
B-12 (mcg)	0	0	0	.02	2.68
Sodium (mg)	4	12	8	18	244
Potassium (mg)	992	0	192	208	702
Calcium (mg)	54	0	6	20	576
Phosphorus (mg)	84	108	4	32	454
Magnesium (mg)	54	0	20	20	48
Iron (mg)	1	0	1.44	.96	0
Zinc	.22	0	.06	.16	2

Two standard servings, for the purposes of this table, include 16 ounces whole milk, 12 ounces brewed coffee, 8 ounces table wine (average red and white), 24 ounces cola, and 16 ounces fresh orange juice.

Adapted from tables in *Food Values of Portions Commonly Used*, 15th edition, by Jean A. T. Pennington. Copyright © 1989 by Jean A. T. Pennington, reprinted by permission of HarperCollinsPublishers, Inc.

TO YOUR HEALTH!

Meanwhile, wine and orange juice have an added value in that they both enhance absorption of iron (and perhaps calcium, phosphorus, magnesium, and zinc) in the rest of the diet. Milk, by contrast, contains no iron and interferes with iron retention from other foods.

To put all of this into perspective, let's refer back for a moment to the RDAs discussed earlier in this chapter. Table A reveals that if a person takes two servings of any of our five beverages, in only two cases will the recommended daily allowance be satisfied (vitamin B-12 in milk and vitamin C in orange juice) and in only a few cases will the beverages account for as much as a third of the RDA (e.g., thiamine in orange juice and riboflavin, folacin, calcium, and phosphorus in milk).

How significant are these contributions? Obviously they do not add much to most people's diets. A better perspective comes from asking a different question: How many American adults depend on the beverage portion of their diets to satisfy nutritional needs? With rare exceptions, the solid portion of our diet satisfies our RDA needs perfectly well (milk's contributions of calcium and phosphorus may be important for some people, especially women, unless their diet includes sufficient amounts of these elements in servings of such foods as cheese or other dairy products).

If it is worth determining what wine contains, it is also worth pointing out what wine *does not* contain: It has no fat or cholesterol and relatively little sodium (relatively more potassium). For those watching their cholesterol intake and for people whose high blood pressure is made

WINE AND NUTRITION

worse by salt intake, this is especially important. For anyone concerned with his or her fat intake, this is also something to be taken into account, as we shall see.

Wine, Calories, and Obesity

For most moderate drinkers, the primary problem is not nutrition but excess calories. Thus wine's greatest impact may be that two servings, regardless of nutritional content, will add to an already calorie-rich diet.*

Scientists disagree, however, about just how many calories an alcohol-containing drink actually provides. Using the standard laboratory techniques, alcohol will give about seven calories per gram (compared with four calories per gram for carbohydrates and nine per gram for fats). However, laboratory measurements do not always predict biological reality, and alcohol in the human body does not create the same number of calories that it does in a lab. As it turns out, individuals who consume a high proportion of their daily required caloric intake from alcohol are likely to lose or maintain weight rather than gain it.**

*According to dietary surveys, about 4–6 percent of total caloric intake in this country comes from alcohol. However, this figure represents an average (teetotalers obviously consume no calories from alcohol, while alcoholics typically get 50 percent or more of their calories from alcohol), and the moderately active, medium-sized man who drinks two glasses a day consumes about 6–8 percent of daily calories from wine. For comparison's sake, we might note that sugar has no nutritional value other than adding calories and typically accounts for some 20 percent of the American diet!

**Given diets of equal caloric content, numerous studies demonstrate that drinkers tend to be less obese than abstainers. Heaviest drinkers tend to have the lowest "body masses," especially for women. Other studies show that moderate drinkers, with higher calorie intake than nondrinkers, weigh about the

Though scientists are still debating what these facts mean for the light, regular drinker, most evidence suggests that alcohol provides an efficient source of immediate energy. And though no one can precisely predict the percent of unused energy the body will store as fat, the amount should be well below the seven calories per gram associated with wine in experiments.

There is another important factor to consider when looking at wine and calories. Substantial evidence now indicates that obesity does not result so much from consuming excessive calories as it does from consuming foods with a high ratio of fat to carbohydrate. (Each body must also undergo sufficient physical activity to burn up calories consumed.) Thus, increasingly, scientists believe that it is not the number of calories consumed per se—obese people do not necessarily consume more calories for their weight than do lean individuals—but the number of those calories derived from fatty foods. Obviously, calories from moderate amounts of wine would contribute significantly less to obesity than equal numbers of calories from, say, butter and oils, meat, nuts, milk, and other fat-containing or fried foods.

Alcohol as a Toxin

In recent years there have been many allegations from advocates of "healthy living" and others that alcohol is an unnatural toxin, a substance that contaminates the otherwise

---

same as nondrinkers. The heaviest drinkers tend to be underweight, though presumably from nutritional deficiencies associated with alcoholism. But no nutritional deficiencies have been linked to light regular alcohol consumption.

inviolable temple of the human body. This simply is not so. Alcohols occur naturally in many of the foods these same people advocate as healthy. For example, yeasts, which are naturally present in fruit and juices, cause fermentation when either the fruit or its juice sits for any length of time, thus producing alcohol in many "natural" fruit products. The human stomach also produces alcohol, up to an ounce or so daily, by the action of bacteria and other microorganisms working on the starches and sugars that course through our gastrointestinal tract. Furthermore, the design of our body allows it to process alcohol with even greater simplicity than it does sugars, fats, and proteins because alcohol requires only one enzyme, alcohol dehydrogenase (a very important substance for our discussion that we will come back to later). Generally speaking, most naturally produced alcohol does not reach the brain because it is produced slowly, absorbed from the gut into the bloodstream, and travels directly to the liver, which processes it into energy before reaching the general circulation.

Of course, at high levels of consumption alcohol can be toxic to human tissue, but we also know that virtually any foodstuff can be toxic at some level of ingestion. Whether in a test tube or in the human body, it is clear that what can nurture human tissue at low concentrations can destroy the same tissue at high concentrations. The potential for toxicity varies from substance to substance and to some degree from person to person; however, no scientific evidence suggests that any common beverage—whether wine, milk, orange juice, coffee, or cola—has significant, lasting toxicity to human tissue at light, regular levels of consumption, that is, one or two standard servings a day.

Alcohol and Diabetes

Diabetes is a metabolic disorder that affects 11 million Americans, and whose most prominent characteristic is an alteration in blood sugar concentration. The two common forms of this disease are insulin-dependent and non-insulin-dependent diabetes. Though alteration in diet has been the foundation of diabetes management for hundreds, perhaps thousands, of years, a consensus about what the optimum dietary management might be remains elusive. Recommendations concerning the ideal proportions of fat and carbohydrates in diabetic diets have fluctuated dramatically over the past two centuries.

Today, scientists favor a high-carbohydrate, low-fat, high-fiber diet and advocate weight loss for the obese as well as restricting the total calorie intake. If these goals can be met, and the diabetic's general condition remains stable, diabetics need not forgo wine. In fact, light, regular wine consumption appears to reduce cardiovascular risk (see chapter 2), to which diabetics are particularly vulnerable. Also, the body burns alcohol without consuming insulin, thereby sparing this vital hormone while providing energy for diabetics.

Milk provides a useful counterpoint to wine in its impact on diabetes. Studies in Canada and Finland suggest that cows' milk triggers diabetes in children who are genetically predisposed to diabetes. As a result, the famous pediatrician

WINE AND NUTRITION

Benjamin Spock reversed his decades-old position encouraging the use of cows' milk, and the American Association of Pediatrics publicly recommended that cows' milk not be used during the first year of life. Compared with consumption of milk, light, regular wine consumption can be seen as neutral or even potentially therapeutic in persons with diabetes or with a predisposition toward diabetes.

THE BOTTOM LINE

In light of what we have learned so far, let's take another look at the questions posed at the beginning of this chapter:

1. *Do wine drinkers consume "empty calories"?* The answer here depends upon how one defines the terms and what the standard of comparison might be. Within the strictest of definitions, the answer is no. Although when compared to beverages like milk and orange juice, wine appears lacking, it does contain nutrients, and next to coffee and cola, it fares quite well.

However, we might say that the real answer is that the question is misleading: No one advocates consuming any of these beverages as an exclusive source of nutrients. Studies show that 75 percent of wine drinkers consume their beverage in the home and 82 percent of this drinking accompanies meals. Also, when consumers drink wine away from home, the majority do so in restaurants, again with meals. Thus, because it regularly accompanies meals, wine does not carry the burden of satisfying a great number of the body's nutritional needs.

TO YOUR HEALTH!

2. *Does wine make any nutritional contribution to the standard diet?* As we have seen, the answer is yes, albeit a relatively small one. Compared with sugar, for example, the standard ingredient in most sweets we consume, wine seems relatively plentiful in nutrients. Compared with certain other foodstuffs, wine is low in nutrients.

But again, the question is misleading because it does not address the entire issue: In addition to the modest amount of nutrients wine contains, it enhances the absorption of a number of minerals, including iron and calcium, a capacity that could be important in individuals who are deficient in these factors. The alcohol in wine clearly plays an important and beneficial role in lipid metabolism (see chapter 2) and may also be beneficial in fat digestion, though scientists have not yet determined in what way and to what degree.

3. *How much does light, regular wine consumption contribute to major nutritional problems?* No evidence exists that light, regular wine consumption in any way causes or contributes to any major nutritional problem. In fact, when compared with other common foodstuffs in the standard diet, table wine fares quite well. Low in salt and sugar and containing no fat, wine helps the body process fat contained in the rest of the meal.

Wine also appears to contribute little to the number-one national nutritional problem, obesity. Not only does wine contribute less fat per calorie than other dietary components, but both demographic and clinical studies suggest that obesity is less a problem among people who drink wine than among others in the population.

4. *Can one do without wine in the diet?* The answer is yes—just as one can do without beef, pork, fish, wheat products, berries, coffee, cola, and so on. Scientists have yet to agree upon a single food item that human beings require for adequate nutrition. On the other hand, no nutritionally based reason exists for excluding light, regular wine consumption from the diet pattern of the average healthy adult.

Chapter 2

Wine and the Heart

Cardiovascular disease (CVD) is the number-one cause of death in every developed country in the world. In the United States, it accounts for nearly 50 percent of the *total* annual mortality rate—nearly as many people die of CVD as die from cancer, accidents, homicides, pneumonia, AIDS, influenza, and all other causes combined.

And, though we have made enormous strides in our understanding of the biggest risk factors for this disease (and we have seen an accompanying dramatic reduction in cardiovascular mortality), nearly one-fourth of the entire living population has at least one form of CVD.

Beyond the obvious personal costs, the amounts spent fighting this illness are also enormous. When you add in the 75 million people who do not die in any given year but who are nonetheless afflicted, the figure becomes astronomical. For example, one million people every year survive heart attacks, and each of these spends an average of seven days in intensive care or a coronary care unit at an average cost per patient of $15,000. At least another 10 million people are hospitalized for one to three days to "rule out" a heart attack after a suspicious episode of chest pain, at an average cost per patient of $3,000. Taking into account cardiac catheterizations, coronary artery bypass surgeries, and coronary angioplasties performed each year, the total yearly cost for CVD-related procedures is at least $100 billion!

Yet these figures do not even begin to estimate the drug therapy and doctor office visit costs for patients with stroke and peripheral vascular disease. They do not include the hundreds of millions of dollars spent annually on drugs that lower blood pressure, regulate heart rate, and enhance the perfusion of cardiac vessels.

The good news is that research over the past forty years has allowed us to develop a much better understanding of the major risk factors for CVD and the markers for premature coronary artery disease, allowing us to reduce our risk for CVD by modifying our lifestyles—primarily through diet and exercise. During this period, we have seen a dramatic reduction in mortality from heart attack and stroke, presumably due to a combination of risk factor reduction and major advances in medical and surgical treatment for CVD: In 1950 the death rate from heart attack and stroke was 316 per 100,000 population; by 1988 that figure had dropped more than 50 percent to 150 per 100,000. Nevertheless, we still see far too many deaths from these diseases. In fact, the growth in population has kept pace with the reduction in mortality, so the actual *number* of deaths per year in the United States has remained nearly constant.

Almost all doctors will agree that diet—lowering our intake of cholesterol and fat-laden foods—is one of the most important parts of any program to manage cardiovascular disease. But there is another very important dietary component that can help in the fight against CVD: wine.

CHOLESTEROL DEPOSITS AND DIET

Early in this century pathologists reported that the coronary arteries of most patients undergoing autopsy had substantial deposits of a peculiar fatty material that narrowed and in many cases completely occluded these vessels. However, they also reported that the coronary vessels of patients who had been heavy drinkers were largely free of these fatty deposits. Composed largely of cholesterol, these "atheromatous lesions" are crucial in the complex process that may ultimately lead to a heart attack, or myocardial infarction (MI), as physicians refer to it.

Another important development came in the 1950s, when pathologists studying the autopsies of GIs killed in the Korean conflict reported that an alarming number of

WINE AND THE HEART

these young men, teenagers in many cases, had early atheromatous disease, and hence were well on their way to the development of premature heart disease. Eventually, through large, carefully controlled research efforts (most notably the ongoing Framingham Study) we have learned that the development of atheromatous deposits depends upon a number of variables, some of which can be greatly influenced by lifestyle—for example, diet, exercise, smoking habits, body weight, and alcohol consumption.

The most direct link between CVD and alcohol intake came in the 1970s, when Dr. Arthur Klatsky, a cardiologist in Oakland, California, noticed that a large number of his heart disease patients were abstainers. Intrigued by the observation, Dr. Klatsky studied the health care records of over 80,000 Kaiser Health Plan patients in northern California and found that men and women who consumed alcoholic beverages were substantially less likely to die of a heart attack than were nondrinkers who were otherwise similar in age and other important variables.

Dr. Klatsky's finding has been replicated dozens of times by numerous scientists using a variety of controls. One such study, published in 1990, specifically looked at the question of whether including former heavy drinkers among current nondrinkers biased Klatsky's results. Instead, the answer confirmed the beneficial effect of light-to-moderate consumption: Excluding former heavy drinkers from the calculations, the results still showed a dramatically reduced mortality risk among moderate drinkers compared with abstainers or heavy drinkers. In fact, in study after study, with diverse populations and other variables being equal or controlled, the light-to-moderate drinking group regularly enjoyed a substantially reduced risk of cardiac death. This benefit also extended beyond the heart to most other forms of cardiovascular disease, including stroke.

In addition to reduced risk of cardiovascular death, another finding that came out of Klatsky's work and others' is that persons who drink fewer than three glasses of wine per day are, as a group, dramatically less likely to require hospitalization for nonfatal cardiovascular problems. Not only is this an important point for those interested in quality of life, it could be a substantial factor in reducing the overall health care costs to society. Remember, several million patients each year survive a heart attack, and millions more are admitted with severe angina or disturbances in the heart rhythm due to coronary artery disease; each requires extraordinarily expensive care.

Just how much of a role can light-to-moderate drinking play in reducing the risk of CVD? Various studies show anywhere from a 20 percent to 40 percent reduction in the risk of death for persons who drink up to three glasses of wine daily. Of course, more is not always better, and these same studies show that persons who drink much more have a higher risk of mortality. Nondrinkers have a certain risk of death; light-to-moderate drinkers have a lower risk of death; while heavy drinkers have the highest risk of death. If we examine the individual studies more closely, we find that the decrease in overall death risk comes entirely from a reduction in risk from CVD. They also show

WINE AND THE HEART

that increasing alcohol consumption does not lead to an increase in cardiovascular risk until a *great* deal is consumed—more than ten drinks per day! Not surprisingly, the relatively high death rate among heavy drinkers (but drinkers who consume fewer than ten drinks per day) is due to noncardiac causes, presumably cirrhosis, traffic accidents, other accidental and violent deaths, cancer, and infectious diseases.*

So, to the extent that wine is drunk at light-to-moderate levels and not associated with increased risk of death due to the noncardiac causes listed above, light-to-moderate wine drinkers can be shown to be a favored group. They enjoy the cardiac benefits of temperate alcohol consumption while not significantly risking death due to alcohol abuse.

ALCOHOL AND CHOLESTEROL

Though the link between moderate wine drinking and reduced cardiovascular risk is now undeniable, scientists are not certain how consumption of wine and other alcoholic

*Just as alcohol can be helpful to the heart in moderate amounts but not at higher levels of consumption, so can fitness and exercise. One recent medical review pointed out that, though "persistent exercise decreases the risk of sudden cardiac death in the long term," sports and exercise "may increase this risk during and immediately after exertion." Another article summed it up as follows: "prudent, regular exercise protects a population against heart disease, but sudden unwise exertion can kill"—an exact parallel to the cardiac effects of moderate versus excessive use of alcohol. Finally, though alcohol provides protection against all types of cardiovascular deaths, it has been reported that drinkers experience a dramatic 50 percent reduction in sudden cardiac death, the most common and most frightening form.

beverages exerts this protective effect upon the heart. Likewise, it remains unclear whether the choice of alcohol matters. There are some strong studies that suggest the cardioprotective effect is uniquely due to wine and that special constituents in wine explain this action, but scientists generally agree that the agent likely to be responsible for most of the cardiac protection is alcohol itself. The most likely basis for alcohol's protective action on the heart and blood vessels is the complex way that alcohol influences fat metabolism. Before we take a look at this process, however, we need to look at the way fats are carried in the bloodstream.

Most of the cholesterol in the bloodstream occurs in a form known as low-density lipoprotein cholesterol, or LDL. It is this LDL that we generally think of when we think of the ill effects of cholesterol: High levels mean an increased risk of coronary artery disease and heart attack. A smaller but variable portion of the total cholesterol in the blood appears as high-density lipoproteins, or HDL. HDL is sometimes referred to as the "good cholesterol." Patients with high blood concentrations of HDL have a markedly reduced risk of coronary artery disease and heart attack. The other main fatty substance in the blood occurs as triglycerides, which appear mainly as very-low-density lipoproteins, or VLDL. Doctors believe that, except in certain lipid disorders or when they are dramatically elevated, triglycerides play a minor role in the start of coronary artery disease.

The most important variable is the *ratio* of HDL to LDL. Simply put, higher ratios deliver a protective effect, and lower ratios correspond to premature disease.

WINE AND THE HEART

Although most physicians have been aware of these facts for several years, until recently the general public's focus has been on total cholesterol.

Nevertheless, physicians, educators, the American Heart Association, and others have succeeded in teaching the public that a high blood cholesterol level correlates with a strong risk for symptomatic coronary artery disease. In the past, as the public awareness of this relationship grew, people began to pay attention to their lifestyles in ways they never did before. In the 1980s it became fashionable to reduce our intake of red meat, and many even adopted a vegetarian diet. People cut down on heavy sauces, cream, and butter; the advertising slogan "no cholesterol" appeared on various food products. Moreover, the growing awareness that risk factors for CVD include a sedentary lifestyle and obesity led legions of Americans to abandon their sedentary behavior in favor of regular exercise, hoping to lower their cholesterol and hence their cardiovascular disease risk.

When dietary changes, aerobic exercise, and attempts to lose weight do not lead to a satisfactory reduction in overall cholesterol, doctors often start patients on one of a range of cholesterol-lowering drugs. These drugs, Mevacor, Lopid, Atromid-S, Questran, Lorelco, Colestid, and others certainly work to lower cholesterol, but they are expensive and their use is so recent that we do not yet know whether they will be free of long-term negative consequences. For example, Mevacor may cause liver abnormalities and muscle damage, and Lopid may cause heartburn, belching, bloating, and a greater likelihood of forming gallstones. Niacin, although the least expensive of the group, can cause severe sensations of feeling flushed and warm, itching, upset stomach, darker skin color, and other problems. Recent work even suggests a marked increase in mortality from cancer and from suicide, homicide, and other violent causes among individuals subjected to cholesterol-lowering interventions.

In contrast, moderate daily amounts of alcohol will quickly lead to a significant increase in HDL cholesterol, producing a favorable HDL/LDL ratio, and it will also bring long-term CVD benefits. And because the benefits of the increased HDL ratio presumably work by retrieving cholesterol deposits from arterial walls and transporting them to the liver where they are further metabolized, it appears that even a person who already has significant cholesterol deposits in blood vessels may reverse at least a portion of the damage done by an earlier unhealthy diet and lifestyle.

Nevertheless, though experts tend to agree in recommending that we avoid high-fat foods and seek out low-fat foods, they have much more difficulty in agreeing on specific foods to recommend. Some recent reports suggest that diets high in calcium and/or vitamin C and/or potassium convey a cardiac benefit, but we are far from a consensus on any of these items. Fish, which beneficially affects the HDL/LDL ratio, has come out very well in numerous studies, but no official body tells us to eat a specific number of servings each week. (In fact, the American Heart Association's major recommendation regarding fish is to tell us to limit consumption: Fish and meat are combined in a food group that includes poultry, legumes, nuts, and eggs, and we are advised to eat no more than two servings a day from the entire group.) Oats and oat bran have also been found to lower cholesterol, but as a specific part of an ideal diet their use remains controversial. So, when cardiologists or dietitians recommend a "heart-wise" diet, they usually focus first on limiting total dietary fat intake and then secondarily on limiting foods that are high in cholesterol or saturated fats.

Alcohol is clearly a subject that is too charged politically in the contemporary environment for groups of conservative scientists to recommend, yet no single dietary component has been so favorably ranked in so many studies concerning cardiovascular mortality or in regard to HDL/LDL effects. For example, as part of a discussion of various dietary manipulations and recommendations, a 1991 *New England Journal of Medicine* editorial observed that "the only dietary factor consistently associated with the risk of coronary heart disease in epidemiological studies is alcohol, which apparently exerts its powerful protective effect at least in part by raising levels of HDL cholesterol." The editorial went on to recommend a glass of red zinfandel "if the urge for an occasional meatball becomes irresistible!"

THE FRENCH PARADOX

Late in 1991 reports from French and American scientists added yet another example to the growing body of data supporting the health advantages of the daily glass of wine. Reported in the popular press as "the French paradox," the phenomenon concerns the very low incidence of heart disease among the French despite a lifestyle characterized by a high-fat diet (much higher even than most Americans'), very little in the way of regular exercise, and widespread cigarette smoking (which is known to be a strong independent risk factor for the development of cardiovascular disease). These scientists attributed the low incidence of heart disease among the French to their daily consumption of alcohol, particularly red wine, with lunch and dinner.

This so-called French paradox was challenged by many who argued, among other things, that the apparent good health of the French stemmed from their relative "starvation" during World War II, predicting that the new generation of Frenchmen would show a much higher level of cardiovascular ill health. This argument was refuted, however, when further analysis of the data, excluding persons older than fifty, still confirmed a lower incidence of heart disease among the French.

Though the data seem to point to alcohol as the active ingredient in promoting cardiovascular health, there are at least some suggestions that wine has a special role. First, wine, more particularly red wine, is the main alcoholic beverage in France and in other Mediterranean countries that share a very low cardiovascular mortality. One report described a large study showing the mortality from twenty-seven Western countries as a function of per capita wine consumption: The greater the per capita wine consumption, the lower the overall risk of death due to cardiovascular disease!

Second is the discovery of a substance that occurs naturally in wine and has a powerful effect upon lipid metabolism. This compound, resveratrol, is manufactured in grapes as they mature, apparently as part of the grapes' resistance to fungal infection. When wine ferments, the resveratrol level in the finished wine increases to a level high enough to have a pharmacological effect. Resveratrol in the human body appears to increase HDL levels while lowering overall cholesterol levels.

Finally, the third factor that may explain a unique cardioprotective effect of wine involves a reduction in "platelet adhesiveness." Platelets are abundant elements in our bloodstream that help in forming clots. Unfortunately, when clotting serves no beneficial function, overactive platelets can cause major problems, such as blockage of vital blood vessels in the heart or in the brain.

Aspirin, one of the most important pharmacological tools that doctors have in treating patients at risk for coronary artery blockage, works its magic through platelets. It reduces the adhesiveness of platelets, and even patients taking small doses have a much reduced likelihood of suffering an acute heart attack. But aspirin is not alone in this regard: Wine appears to have a similar effect on platelets. In addition, it has a beneficial impact on blood lipids and atherosclerosis, giving it far broader cardiovascular usefulness than aspirin. Furthermore, a recent study reported that this antiplatelet effect stemmed from tannins and other components that are found in wine but not in other alcoholic beverages.

HYPERTENSION AND DIET

Another important risk factor for the development of cardiovascular disease (and for stroke) is hypertension, or high blood pressure. Hypertension appears to be a disease of affluent, developed countries. Approximately 20 percent of adults over the age of forty in the United States are afflicted, and many persons involved in fighting CVD have argued that hypertension is primarily responsible for our country's high cardiovascular mortality. We spend billions of dollars every year on its detection, treatment, and monitoring.

To understand the effect of high blood pressure on the heart, visualize the following: Our body demands a certain minimum blood flow to nourish its tissues—roughly five quarts per minute in the average adult at rest. Naturally, when we exert ourselves the flow must increase to meet the metabolic demands of our tissues. We have complex control mechanisms to assure that blood flow meets these demands: At maximum physical exertion, it may increase by as much as six times the resting level! Of course, all blood flow is due to the pumping action of the heart, so blood pressure is determined by cardiac output, on the one hand, and the resistance to flow through the arteries, on the other. Therefore our blood pressure can go up with increasing output and/or with increasing resistance to flow.

The higher the pressure in the arteries, the greater the pressure the heart has to generate in order to pump blood through them. The higher the pressure the heart has to generate, the stronger and more massive it has to be and the more work it has to perform. But the heart muscle itself requires blood flow to obtain oxygen and nutrients in the same way that other tissues do, and the more work the heart performs, the more oxygen it needs. If the coronary artery is narrowed or blocked, the heart muscle will not get enough oxygen. If the lack of oxygen is substantial, a portion of the muscle may die, resulting in myocardial infarction (literally, "heart muscle death")—a heart attack.

Even if the blockage is not so severe as to cause a heart attack, however, damage may be done. The heart beats an average of about 115,000 times every day, 42 million times per year. If the heart must beat against a higher pressure, it is no surprise that it will not last as long as it would pumping against a lower pressure.

What causes high blood pressure? In some people it can be explained by specific diseases, but most hypertensive individuals suffer from what we call "essential hypertension," which means only that the specific cause is unknown. We do know that because hypertension has a tendency to run in families, heredity clearly plays a role in its development. Gender also seems to be a factor: More men than women have elevated blood pressure in preretirement years, though more women over sixty-five have hypertension than men of comparable age. Race, too, is important: Hypertension afflicts more blacks than whites, with blacks getting the disease younger, in greater numbers, and with more severe consequences.

As for the effect of diet, its part is not a simple one. We know that people who are obese (i.e., more than 30 percent above ideal weight) have a greater risk of hypertension than people of normal weight. We also know that though not everyone is affected equally, the single aspect of diet most likely to make hypertension worse is excessive salt intake. (When excessive salt is taken in, the body responds by increasing all the fluids outside the cells, including blood. At the same time, it tries to eliminate more salt in the urine. This increase in fluid causes an increase in blood pressure in salt-sensitive individuals that in turn causes an increased load on the heart.)*

As for the effect of wine on hypertension, the most widely accepted view is that *excessive* alcohol consumption leads to an increase in blood pressure.

It is true that alcoholics have a high incidence of hypertension. And though some have argued that alcohol's effect upon blood pressure is a cumulative one and that even light-to-moderate consumption over the long haul may lead

---

It is worth pointing out that, although salt-sensitive hypertensives are a huge group of people (as many as 18 percent of whites and 37 percent of blacks), the government, which aggressively requires warning labels on alcoholic beverages, has never suggested warning labels on foods such as salted crackers and chips, pretzels, pickles, soy sauce, sauerkraut, luncheon meats, and so on. Even at moderate consumption levels, these and other high-salt items may present a far greater health hazard to far more people than alcohol does.

to the development of hypertension, the best studies show that light-to-moderate drinkers have blood pressures that are similar to or lower than those of abstainers. In fact, many studies show a J-shaped curve, in which light-to-moderate drinkers have lower blood pressures than abstainers or heavy drinkers.

Though the mechanism for alcohol's effect upon blood pressure is still only conjecture, the effect among heavy drinkers appears to be real and probably explains the increased risk of stroke and cardiac disease in the heaviest drinkers. (In addition to being an independent risk factor for the development of coronary artery disease, hypertension is the dominant risk factor for stroke.)* But the data concerning alcohol consumption and the risk of stroke are mixed. One large study published in 1990 showed a reduction in risk for all types of stroke in patients consuming light-to-moderate amounts of alcohol. Other data show light-to-moderate drinkers have a decreased risk of ischemic stroke but a somewhat increased risk of hemorrhagic stroke.

Obviously, we must look at these facts carefully and weigh several considerations. For example, we must con-

---

*Stroke *is the general term used to describe the sudden loss of function in any part of the brain due to an event occurring in a cerebral vessel, usually an artery. There are two kinds of stroke, ischemic and hemorrhagic. In an ischemic stroke, sometimes referred to as a "dry" stroke, there is sudden cessation of blood flow to a part of the brain, resulting in "ischemia," or oxygen starvation of the brain tissue involved. If this ischemia is prolonged, the brain tissue dies; this is referred to as an infarction. In a hemorrhagic or "wet" stroke, a blood vessel bleeds into the brain or the space around the brain known as the subarachnoid space. Either of these events can prove fatal depending upon the extent of the bleeding or the size and location of the ischemic brain tissue.*

TO YOUR HEALTH!

sider any negative health effects of alcohol in light of the strong health benefits seen with light-to-moderate drinking. Though heavy drinkers have a higher risk of hypertension and stroke than do nondrinkers or light-to-moderate drinkers, light-to-moderate drinkers enjoy a significantly better mortality risk than do abstainers. Hence, any effect upon blood pressure does not translate into an increased risk of death for light-to-moderate drinkers.

CARDIAC ARRHYTHMIAS AND DIET

One additional aspect of CVD that we have not yet discussed concerns cardiac arrhythmias. A cardiac arrhythmia is simply a disturbance in the heart rate or regularity. These disturbances can range from imperceptible and benign changes to catastrophic and even fatal events.

The most common arrhythmias involve variations in heart rate, or the rapidity with which the heart beats. Virtually everyone is familiar with situations in which the heart beats faster than what is regarded, strictly speaking, as normal, for example, in times of emotional stress, fear, anticipation, anxiety, and anger. Though physicians label 60 to 100 beats per minute as "normal," the healthy heart can stand a much wider range, and very rapid rates (up to 180 beats per minute and more in trained athletes) are usually well tolerated during times of excitement or physical exertion. It is only when these high rates are persistent, occur at rest, or afflict people with diseased hearts that they become cause for concern. Certain irregularities in heart rhythm are also common and do not necessarily indicate the presence of any disease or potential disability. Those that originate in the upper part of the heart (the atria) occur in all age groups and are usually found in the absence of heart disease; however, certain heart diseases predispose a patient to these irregularities and can make their presence more worrisome. These atrial irregularities can be precipitated by emotion, fatigue, and medications (e.g., over-the-counter decongestants or asthma medications), as well as by dieting and fasting. Specific food items such as coffee, chocolate, and alcoholic beverages also can be factors.

Irregularities originating in the lower part of the heart (the ventricles) are the most common arrhythmias, both in health and in disease. Some normal people are particularly prone to extra beats in the ventricles, but these can remain asymptomatic even over many years. Ventricular arrhythmias may also result from heart disease and can be a worrisome sign of electrically unstable heart tissue. In both health and disease, such irregularities can be brought about or made worse by reduced oxygen, by alterations in potassium or calcium intake, by various medications, and by such foods as caffeine-containing beverages, chocolate, and alcohol. Caffeine, for example, when taken by nonusers, can cause increased heart rate, produce extra heartbeats, and even raise cholesterol and blood pressure. However, most people develop a tolerance to caffeine, and the clear majority of people have no cardiac abnormalities when drinking normal amounts. In fact, there are even studies purporting to show that blood pressure goes *down* with increased coffee consumption.

The same pattern holds true for alcoholic beverages in general and red wine in particular. Though some people have what doctors like to term "idiosyncratic reactions" and develop palpitations or cardiac irregularities after drinking red wine (or other alcoholic beverages), this response seems to differ with individuals and does not represent a risk for the population in general. Obviously, people who know that wine makes their heart beat rapidly or irregularly will wish to avoid it.

WEIGHING THE RISKS

As we have seen, the single greatest risk to life and health in developed countries is cardiovascular disease—nothing else comes close. If you want to extend not only your life but your healthy years, you owe it to yourself to look after your heart and blood vessels. Lifestyle is clearly an important factor in caring for your circulatory system, and, though some issues may be controversial, a few medical facts stand out:

1. Cigarette smoking has a universal and overwhelmingly negative impact upon the incidence of heart disease and stroke. If you have not stopped smoking already, you should do so now.

2. Maintaining a reasonably normal body weight—certainly within 30 percent of the ideal weight for your height

and age group—and keeping cholesterol levels within normal ranges are both important. Regular exercise is also helpful in the long run; however, strenuous exercise that requires sudden bursts of exertion carries a definite cardiac risk.

3. Beyond these measures, the medical literature to date suggests that the single most useful step you can take to protect your heart is to make regular, light-to-moderate amounts of alcohol, especially wine, a part of your diet. It may not be politic to say so in public, but anyone who looks carefully and critically at contemporary medical literature can hardly come to any other conclusion.

For all the caution of scientific committees and governmental advisory boards, and in spite of the strident rhetoric of the antialcohol community, no other food or beverage comes close to achieving the positive effect of the consumption of light-to-moderate amounts of alcohol, especially wine, on cardiac health. In fact, if you examine health effects solely in terms of cardiovascular impact, the evidence thus far is massively in favor of wine.

If you are among the millions of Americans who enjoy a glass of wine with meals and who do not experience any of the adverse effects or risks discussed in this or other chapters, you can take comfort in knowing that the wine you drink clearly lowers your risk of both fatal and nonfatal cardiac disease. Whatever alcohol's variable and idiosyncratic effects on blood pressure and cardiac rhythms, the bottom line is that wine helps the vast majority of light-to-moderate consumers live longer lives with a lower incidence of cardiac disease.

TO YOUR HEALTH!

If you do not do so already, should you start drinking wine to reduce your chances of heart disease? The answer here is more complicated, and you must carefully balance risks and benefits. However, if you are not at risk of becoming a problem drinker, if you do not belong to a family or ethnic group at high risk of alcoholism, if you have not had trouble in the past with prescription or recreational drugs, and if you are not at special risk because of attributes and conditions discussed in this or other chapters, then light, regular wine drinking as part of your diet certainly is worth considering.

Of course, these recommendations are not meant to suggest that wine is any kind of panacea. As we mentioned earlier, the most effective means of correcting a cardiovascular problem is not through what you *add* to your diet but what you subtract or limit. So, if your diet is rich in fats and cholesterol, if you smoke or do not exercise, it is more important to alter those habits than to rely on alcohol to compensate for the negative aspects of your lifestyle. Light, regular wine consumption is a useful component of a heart-wise lifestyle, but it is by no means the only component. Good heart sense requires healthy living.

Chapter 3

Wine and the Digestive Tract

Wine has been called "the most ancient dietary beverage and the most important medicinal agent in continuous use throughout the history of the world," yet many regard it as primarily a poison, responsible for various cancers of the digestive tract, as well as inflammatory and scarring diseases such as cirrhosis of the liver. Indeed alcohol can impact every tissue throughout the gastrointestinal tract, but does the individual who enjoys wine with meals risk gastritis, pancreatitis, ulcer disease, and liver problems? And how does the effect of light, regular wine drinking upon the GI tract compare with that of other foods and beverages?

Though it is true that alcohol in high concentrations—40 percent ethanol or higher, such as is found in distilled spirits—can harm the tissues of the mouth, throat, and stomach, the concentration of alcohol in wine, even fortified wines, is not great enough to be significantly irritating. This effect of chemical irritation can cause the sensation of burning we often experience with "straight" alcohol. At times, these inflammatory conditions can cause uncomfortable symptoms that interfere with normal living and lead individuals to seek medical care. In the case of esophagitis and gastritis, inflammation of the esophagus and stomach, life-threatening bleeding may result. Moreover, alcohol's direct irritant effect plays a role in the development of cancer of these tissues, particularly if accompanied by tobacco smoke or other irritants. Once again, however, the alcohol concentration in wine is not enough to have an effect.

The real effect of wine on our digestive tract occurs in the process of digestion itself. This begins even before we start to drink. The smell, sight, or even the very thought of any food or drink stimulates the flow of saliva and prepares the stomach and intestines for action. When wine actually enters the mouth, the flow of saliva increases at once, reaching its peak about ten minutes after drinking, and the increased salivation continues for at least an hour with or without additional food. This is an important part of the digestive process because saliva contains the enzyme salivary amylase, which begins the breakdown of starches and complex sugars and lubricates the esophagus for swallowing.

WINE AND THE DIGESTIVE TRACT

Another enzyme secreted in the mouth in response to the acid stimulus of wine begins the breakdown of fatty acids.

One additional benefit of these enzymes and other salivary secretions stimulated by wine may be dental health: It appears that they reduce plaque formation and inhibit decay-causing bacteria. But let's look now at wine's effect on the next level of digestion.

THE STOMACH

In order to digest the food it receives, the stomach maintains a very acidic environment. Specialized cells actually secrete a solution of hydrochloric acid that is concentrated enough to burn most biological tissues. In order to contain the acid without burning its own lining and ultimately destroying itself, the stomach differs from the rest of the gut in that it is nearly impermeable to water and only very minimally affected by the acid it secretes. This characteristic is known as the "gastric mucosal barrier." Although we do not fully understand how it works, this mechanism serves to protect the stomach from the acid. Nevertheless, certain substances can damage the gastric mucosal barrier, including aspirin, such foods as hot peppers, and ethanol in concentrations greater than 20 percent.*

*Early investigations of the effects of alcohol on the digestive system focused on the stomach. In one especially famous series of observations, the nineteenth-century physician William Beaumont described a man who had been shot in the abdomen: The gunshot wound left him with an accidental gastrostomy (literally, a hole in the stomach), which allowed direct observation of the stomach. Dr. Beaumont found that alcohol in high concentrations will

When the barrier breaks, the stomach lining loses its impermeability, allowing deep penetration of acid into submucosal tissues. The acid in turn stimulates local nerve networks and causes the strong contractions and sometimes severe pain associated with ulcers. Unfortunately, the mucosa also secretes increased quantities of protein-digesting enzymes and releases histamine, which stimulates further acid secretion in addition to triggering a series of inflammatory events with swelling and injury to the tiny blood vessels called capillaries. The whole process may become a vicious cycle and result in massive bleeding as the stomach literally digests itself.

Because alcohol in concentrations of 40 percent and greater so clearly causes injury to the lining of the stomach, scientists now routinely use alcohol in animal experiments to study the self-defense mechanisms of the gastric mucosa. They have found that low concentrations of alcohol, such as is found in wine, stimulate acid secretion but do not injure the mucosal lining. Nevertheless, a preexisting mucosal injury or ingestion of another, more toxic substance may predispose the stomach to injury.

Interestingly, concentrations of alcohol of less than 20 percent, about the concentration found in fortified wines, actually can protect the lining of the duodenum (the first

---

directly and quickly damage the lining of the stomach, the so-called gastric mucosa. Since then a good deal of work has replicated and confirmed these findings. Another finding has shown that much of the stomach's self-protective effect appears to be due to a naturally occurring local hormone called prostaglandin. Aspirin and ibuprofen are prostaglandin inhibitors and thus increase the risk of gastritis, duodenitis, and gastrointestinal bleeding.

WINE AND THE DIGESTIVE TRACT

portion of the small intestine) from inflammations associated with subsequent exposure to higher doses of alcohol. As in so many other cases, a substance that can cause harm at high doses may actually have a therapeutic effect in low concentrations.

Many people, including some doctors, mistakenly believe that alcohol causes ulcer disease. It does not. Ulcer disease occurs more commonly in cirrhosis patients, whether or not the cirrhosis is alcohol related. In other words, though we tend to think of someone suffering from cirrhosis as an alcoholic, this is not necessarily the case (as we will see later), and cirrhosis due to hepatitis B is just as likely to be associated with ulcers as cirrhosis due to alcohol. Certainly, light, regular wine drinking does not cause an increased risk of gastric or duodenal ulcers. However, most doctors do recommend that individuals with active ulcer disease give up all alcohol.

One last note of interest: Scientists have recently discovered a stomach enzyme that greatly influences alcohol metabolism: gastric alcohol dehydrogenase, or ADH, previously found only in the liver. Most people appear to metabolize a significant amount of alcohol via this enzyme—about 20 percent—before it can be absorbed by the stomach. The presence of such a preabsorptive metabolism helps to explain some of the enormous variation in peak blood alcohol levels (discussed in more detail in later chapters). Any condition that slows the stomach from emptying itself allows more time for the action of ADH, reduces the amount of alcohol absorbed, hence also the peak alcohol level in the blood. As we explain in chapter 5, reduced activity of gastric ADH may partially account for women's reduced tolerance to alcohol.

THE LIVER AND CIRRHOSIS

Cirrhosis of the liver is a disease that results from repeated liver injury, causing cells to die and be replaced initially by fat and ultimately by scar tissue. As most of us are aware, it is a serious and often life-threatening condition. This is so because the liver is such a vital organ and plays a key role in so many metabolic processes. Among other tasks, the liver performs most of the transformations of nutrients and chemicals in our diet. It "detoxifies" many potentially toxic chemicals and pharmaceuticals that cannot be excreted in the urine, including alcohol. In fact, at least 75 percent of the alcohol we consume is metabolized in the liver (via the same enzyme used in the stomach, ADH).* The liver also controls lipid and steroid metabolism and participates importantly in sugar and protein metabolism, allowing the individual to maintain a steady level of such nutrients in the bloodstream. The liver plays a central role in fat metabolism: It controls the levels of LDL and HDL cholesterol as well as triglycerides, and it manufactures bile, which emulsifies fats to render them more readily absorbed by the gut.

*Interestingly, exposure to alcohol causes the liver to greatly increase its capacity to metabolize alcohol and other drugs. This happens through a process known as "enzyme induction," which results in a markedly enhanced activity of a specific enzyme system, cytochrome P450.

But when it is substantially scarred, the liver cannot function normally. Such scarring leads to varying degrees of failure and causes such problems as weight loss, fatigue, diarrhea, and disordered thinking, among others. Hepatic coma, meaning "liver coma," eventually ensues, followed by death, unless some other complication of cirrhosis kills first.

Not only does the scarred liver lose many of its vital metabolic capabilities, the scarring will eventually block, partially or completely, the low pressure portal vein that delivers blood into the liver directly from the intestines. The increased pressure in the portal system causes health problems for cirrhosis patients, including fluid accumulation in the abdomen (a dramatically swollen belly is typical of cirrhosis sufferers) and dilation of blood vessels in the lower esophagus with the potential for massive bleeding. Cirrhotics also have a high incidence of other potentially lethal complications such as peritonitis, bacteremia (bacterial invasion of the bloodstream), and infected heart valves.

Cirrhosis is most often associated with heavy drinking, and indeed it is one of the greatest and most common health dangers due to alcoholism. In fact, public health authorities long regarded the incidence of mortality due to liver cirrhosis as a key indicator of alcohol abuse in our society because most cases occur in heavy drinkers. However, it is also true that among heavy drinkers, the majority never show evidence of liver cirrhosis, which would indicate that certain individuals are more susceptible than others to this disease. Moreover, though excessive drinking can cause cirrhosis, the condition may also come from various forms of viral hepatitis or from exposure to other toxic chemicals, such as solvents and some anesthetic agents. In fact, at least 40 percent of liver cirrhosis cases result from causes other than alcohol.

What about wine? Is there an association with liver disease among those who enjoy light, regular wine consumption? Mortality statistics and consumption patterns provide weak but suggestive evidence regarding the risk of wine drinking and liver cirrhosis. Although published reports in the past suggested that wine actually *helped* in the treatment of cirrhotic patients,* doctors today would not recommend any alcohol intake in such patients, because of much more effective modern management techniques. In fact, individuals with cirrhosis or any symptoms of impaired liver function should not drink at all.

Here are some of the facts we know about cirrhosis and wine. In 1974 the annual mortality from cirrhosis in the United States was approximately fifteen per 100,000 of the population. Over the next ten years the mortality due to cirrhosis decreased gradually every year to a level of approximately ten per 100,000 population in 1983, a reduction of about 30 percent. During this same period, the per capita consumption of spirits decreased by 6 percent, but the per capita wine consumption rose 37 percent and beer consumption rose 16 percent.

Carbone at San Francisco General Hospital reported effective treatment of alcoholics with cirrhosis using a combined high-nutrient diet with up to one liter's wine ration per day (J. Clin. Invest. 1957).

WINE AND THE DIGESTIVE TRACT

More precise studies reveal that the volume of alcohol required to produce significant liver injury for most men is quite large, eighty grams per day for fifteen years or more. This corresponds to a daily intake of approximately one liter of wine, a half-pint of whiskey, or eight 12-ounce beers (the threshold for liver injury in women may be as low as half to three-quarters as much). Of course, these high levels of consumption cause other toxic effects, quite apart from the effect on the GI system, and obviously they do not pertain to the normal wine drinker engaged in light, regular wine drinking, who need not worry about cirrhosis.

THE PANCREAS AND THE INTESTINES

Like the liver, the pancreas contributes to the digestive process. At least seven different enzymes as well as the essential hormones involved in the regulation of sugar metabolism come from the pancreas. Wine and a variety of foods strongly stimulate the secretion of pancreatic juices, which persists for at least an hour. However, repeated high doses of alcohol (enough to produce intoxication) often lead to the abrupt development of pancreatitis, a remarkably painful ailment associated with inflammation of the pancreas. Pancreatitis causes severe, unremitting pain and intractable vomiting. It can lead to a dramatic disruption in the normal control of blood sugar levels and can also cause life-threatening disruptions in calcium balance. Although a severe blow to the abdomen can also cause severe pancreatitis, excessive consumption of alcohol is the most common cause.

TO YOUR HEALTH!

Though we can find no evidence that light, regular wine drinking causes pancreatitis initially, most doctors believe that any alcohol intake can cause a recurrence of pancreatitis after the first episode. Therefore, the best advice to anyone who has had an episode of pancreatitis is to avoid drinking any alcoholic beverages.

As for the small and large intestines, little published work has focused on the effects of alcohol on this part of the digestive tract. Our own belief is that there is little positive or negative effect. Obviously if drinking is so excessive that it leads to reduced consumption of dietary fiber, it will very likely contribute to constipation and to the development of hemorrhoids. However, light, regular wine drinking actually produces a salutary effect upon constipation that has been described for decades. One relatively recent report suggests that heavy drinkers, especially if they also smoke, develop colonic polyps more frequently than do nondrinkers. Because colonic polyps may progress to cancer, this result suggests a higher incidence of colon cancer in heavy drinkers. Wine drinkers, by contrast, very likely enjoy some protection from gastrointestinal cancers due to the presence of quercetin in wine (see chapter 4).

RESULTS

Excessive drinking of any alcoholic beverage clearly causes severe gastrointestinal disease, the most devastating being liver damage. However, there does not appear to be any significant gastrointestinal risk associated with light, regular wine drinking, whereas such drinking does provide some beneficial stimulus to the digestive process.

Of course, many common foodstuffs, beverages, and habits strongly contribute to the development of significant GI disorders. Diseases aggravated by common foodstuffs run the spectrum from uncomfortable minor symptoms (stomach pains after several cups of coffee), to life-threatening, catastrophic illness. With wine, as with any other foodstuff, one's own personal medical history must first be taken into account, but, on balance, light, regular wine drinking is a reasonable choice for most generally healthy adults concerned about their gastrointestinal health.

Chapter 4

Cancer

Cancer. This simple word strikes terror into the hearts of people everywhere. Doctors almost always use some code word so they can talk about cancer in polite company or soften the blow when speaking to a patient or family about a diagnosis of cancer. Sometimes patients leave their doctor's office after being told they have a "carcinoma," a "neoplasm," a "metastasis," or a "malignancy" without understanding that each term is an exact synonym for cancer.

Because the prospect of dying from cancer is so abhorrent to most of us, and because a cure seems so elusive, we avidly seek ways to reduce our risk: As a society we often approve the regulation of any substance that shows even the slightest association with an increased cancer risk.

Ironically, however, the greatest risk factor is something we have no control over: age. The likelihood of contracting cancer increases dramatically as we grow older, and by the sixth decade and beyond the risk is high. The more successful we are in avoiding death from accidents, infection, and cardiovascular disease, the more likely it is that we will ultimately die of cancer.

CANCER, CARCINOGENS, AND GENETICS

Although a great deal of research has been done on cancer, its various forms and their causes, much remains shrouded in mystery and controversy. We know, for example, that cancers originate in normal body tissue during cell division (mitosis) and that this is set off by a mutation in the DNA of the parent cell. However, this mutation must occur in a specific part of the DNA strand having to do with control of cell growth, differentiation, or recognition of neighboring cells. Any of a number of factors acting alone or in harmony with other variables can cause such an event.

Except for nerve cells, each and every part of the body gradually replaces itself over and over throughout our lives. Approximately 10 million cells divide every minute in adults. Some tissues replace themselves more frequently, requiring a more rapid pace of cell division, and this feature makes these tissues more susceptible to cancerous transformation. For example, the epithelial tissues lining the gastrointestinal tract turn over very rapidly, and cancers of the GI tract are the most common of human cancers. Certain other tissues are more routinely exposed to carcinogens and thus display a strong tendency to become cancerous, as in the case of lung cancer among smokers.

Of course, cells normally divide in a very predictable, orderly, and controlled way, but occasionally a mutation may cause them to divide abnormally and much more rapidly. It is this rapidly growing tissue that doctors call a tumor. If it does not grow uncontrollably or spread to other parts of the body, the tumor is benign and usually is not removed unless it causes cosmetic or functional impairment due to its size or location. If, however, the tumor invades the surrounding tissues or spreads through the blood or lymph to remote parts of the body and grows wildly there, it is termed malignant, that is, a cancer. Cancers kill people because they do not perform any useful function and they grow to such an extent as to crowd out or destroy normal, productive tissue. Surgery performed early enough, before the malignant cells have a chance to spread or invade surrounding tissue, is the only real cure for most cancers.

Though we do not know why some people get cancer and others do not under the same conditions, we do know that exposure to certain substances puts an individual at high risk of developing cancer. Any substance that makes cancer more likely in people exposed to it is termed a *carcinogen*. Experts believe that carcinogens are of two general types: initiators and promoters. Initiators start the damage to a cell that can lead directly to cancer (unless the body is able to repair the damage). Promoters usually do not directly cause cancer but may interact with a cell already damaged by an initiator to change it into a cancer cell. Cigarette smoke and smokeless tobacco are both very strong initiators.

In addition to exposure to carcinogens, genetics plays a strong role in whether or not a given person will contract certain forms of cancer. Each individual possesses a set of genes (most of which have not been identified) that can be termed *cancer susceptibility* genes. These genes work to influence risk of cancer in a variety of ways, ranging from the way carcinogens are metabolized to the capacity of the immune system to recognize and destroy malignant cells. But here again no hard-and-fast rules apply, and the details by which an individual's inherited genetic material may operate have yet to be worked out. Also, a second class of genes operates in league with the general susceptibility of the individual to cancer. When damaged or altered, these genes, called *oncogenes*, cause the cells in which they are located to become cancerous.

ESTABLISHING CAUSE

Scientists and physicians believe that most cancers are caused by oncogenes through a combination of genetic predisposition plus occupational factors, lifestyle, and exposure to cancer-causing substances. Hence, if I have several relatives with cancer and I also smoke, I am dramatically more likely to get cancer than the average smoker. If several relatives had suffered skin cancer, I would be well advised to stay out of the sun as much as possible.

Because we cannot at present control or alter our genetic background and yet we want desperately to avoid the awful specter of cancer, we work hard and spend enormous amounts of money to identify and avoid exposure to carcinogens. But some readers may be astonished to learn that scientists have a very hard time actually proving that any substance causes cancer *in humans*. This is difficult because substances known to cause cancer in rats or other experimental animals may be harmless in humans.

For example, most of us know that saccharin causes bladder cancer in rats. Because of this finding, even without showing a link to human cancer, the Canadian government and the U.S. Food and Drug Administration banned saccharin in 1977. Although public pressure in support of saccharin eventually forced Congress to lift this ban, by law all products containing saccharin must bear a warning label. In 1992, we learned that the mechanism by which saccharin causes cancer in rats does not exist in humans; hence there is no chance that saccharin causes cancer in humans at all! Still, the warning labels remain in place.

Scientists generally accept a substance as a proven carcinogen if appropriate studies show a strong association with cancer in humans, if animals exposed to the agent develop cancer, and if some plausible mechanism exists by which the agent may be expected to act. When one or more of these features is lacking, experts regard the substance as a possible or "putative" carcinogen. As we shall see, however, even when all three elements coincide, proof of causation remains elusive.

Studies have identified an enormous number of potentially cancer-causing compounds. But to understand some of the difficulties in proving the validity of various risk factors, let us examine one specific type of malignancy, breast cancer.

Among women, this is the most common form of cancer and, after lung cancer, causes more deaths than any other cancer. The overall risk of developing breast cancer among women in the United States has doubled since 1940, and surveys show a steadily increasing incidence. Over a span of eighty-five years, the average life expectancy for women, the current calculated risk for breast cancer in the United States is approximately 11 percent. Unfortunately, many doctors who should know better translate this as indicating that 11 percent of all women will suffer breast cancer. This is simply not so. What this says is that *the statistical likelihood of contracting breast cancer for a population of women all living to age eighty-five is 11 percent—* quite a different statement. This statistic does not take into account the enormous risk differences between populations and does not address the cumulative risk with advancing age. Obviously, then, some women have a much higher risk than others. For example, some women with specific inheritance backgrounds and specific lifestyle patterns are almost certain to get breast cancer, while other women with different genetic backgrounds are very unlikely to get the disease. According to the Surgeon General, *relative risk* may vary by more than a hundredfold. People should understand this enormous naturally occurring risk differential when trying to interpret reports that a particular substance may increase breast cancer risk by 20 or even 50 percent.

A great number of other factors may also be involved: Hormonal balance and oral contraceptives probably figure prominently in the risk for breast cancer, but the picture remains clouded; being underweight before menopause (but being obese after), having large breasts, and being a lesbian (probably because these women are less likely to bear children—among women who never bear children or whose first birth occurs after age twenty-five, breast cancer risk escalates dramatically) are all additional factors.

CANCER, DIET, AND WINE

According to the 1988 *Surgeon General's Report on Health and Nutrition,* diet plays a causative role in at least 35 percent of all cancer deaths, a larger role than any other category of risk. One of the biggest culprits is fat. Animal studies showing fat to be a "promoter" date back to 1930, and this link has been consistently reported in subsequent human studies. However, a great number of other food products have also been reported to cause cancer, including meat protein; eggs; vegetable fat; polyunsaturated fats; and salt-pickled, salt-cured, and smoked foods; as well as certain dietary habits like low fiber intake and deficiencies in

68 such elements as selenium, calcium, vitamin A, vitamin E, and vitamin C.

Not only are specific food items associated with cancer, but our overall caloric intake is also associated strongly with cancer risk in both animal and human studies. This association grows stronger year by year, with many published reports. Similarly, body weight as an indicator for excessive overall food consumption correlates with cancer risk.

How can one weigh the relative contributions of various factors to cancer risk? A summary table from the Surgeon General's report provides some perspective: After dietary considerations, tobacco use follows closely, at 30 percent, with reproductive and sexual behavior involved in an estimated 7 percent. What about alcohol? The best estimate for alcohol was reported as 3 percent—the same as was listed for "geophysical factors"! Despite numbers such as these, many find it all too easy to excoriate alcoholic beverages for any health problem regardless of the risk. Thus, although the American Cancer Society had served wine and cheese at receptions and fund-raisers for years, in the early 1980s it banned the serving of any alcoholic beverage, including wine, at any of its functions. Why? Did someone show that wine causes cancer? Not really.

For many years doctors learned in medical school that heavy drinkers of distilled spirits get certain kinds of cancers much more commonly than do nondrinkers. For example, cancer of the tongue, the larynx, the esophagus, the stomach, and the pancreas are all more common in drinkers of spirits. Also, national epidemiological studies from European countries revealed an increased incidence of cancer among individuals involved in the manufacture and distribution of alcoholic beverages.

In the 1970s and early 1980s several strong reports underlined the association of heavy drinking with oral and other gastrointestinal cancers, including cancers of the larynx, esophagus, stomach, and pancreas. The accumulating evidence linking alcohol consumption with cancer caught the attention of the American Cancer Society, which did not want to be portrayed as hypocritical. A strong lobby within the organization pushed to eliminate alcoholic beverages, even wine and cheese receptions, from their activities, although wine drinking was not specifically associated with increased cancer risk.

The argument for this ban was based upon the concept of "active ingredients": If the active ingredient in spirits and beer is alcohol, and if drinking spirits and beer leads to cancer, drinking anything else that contains alcohol must lead to cancer also. According to this logic, wine, although never separately implicated as a cancer-causing agent, must also be a carcinogen because it contains alcohol.

At about the same time, the Center for Science in the Public Interest and Mothers Against Drunk Driving, as well as other groups, actively lobbied to eliminate all public drinking. They pushed particularly to eliminate drinking in settings that they thought could somehow lend a sense of respectability to drinking.

In the face of this kind of pressure, with data accumulating that alcohol in high concentration causes cancer (actually, most experts believe that alcohol as a carcinogen is not an initiator, but a promoter), the ACS capitulated.

It was at this same time that Dr. Klatsky and others published data illustrating the cardioprotective effect of alcohol (see chapter 2). Thus the American Heart Association continued to pour wine at its functions and fund-raisers, buoyed by the breaking wave of evidence that drinking can be healthful. For though cancer now accounts for upwards of 20 percent of all deaths annually in the United States, the leading cause of death by far is still heart disease. According to the American Heart Association, heart disease is responsible for over 50 percent of all female deaths in the United States and 40 percent or more of all male deaths. We may be terrified of cancer, but we are dying of heart disease.

Although earlier studies showed either no relationship or a very weak relationship between alcohol consumption and breast cancer, a 1987 *New England Journal of Medicine* article reported a higher incidence of breast cancer in women who drink alcoholic beverages. The authors reported that even moderate amounts of alcohol increased the risk of breast cancer measurably. However, in this study, breast cancer risk rose in those drinking beer or spirits but not in wine drinkers. The authors ignored this finding, though, because the reduction in risk among wine drinkers was not statistically significant and did not fit the preconception that alcohol causes cancer.

Since those reports, several more recent publications have disputed the association of moderate alcohol use with breast cancer. Some studies found that moderate consumption of alcohol may actually *decrease* the risk of various kinds of cancers. For example, an American Cancer Society study published in 1990 showed a decreased risk of skin and gastrointestinal cancers in moderate drinkers, and a study by the U.S. Department of Health and Human Services involving several thousand women showed no correlation with breast cancer for women consuming fewer than twenty-two drinks per week! Another ACS study reported a significant decrease in overall cancer deaths among men consuming fewer than two drinks daily, and a *New England Journal of Medicine* article showed increased colon cancer in beer drinkers but not in wine drinkers. Reports published in 1993 linking moderate alcohol consumption to increased breast cancer risk must be interpreted cautiously.

CANCER PREVENTION AND WINE

Humans consume an astonishing array of organic and inorganic substances. Logic suggests that if exposure to some chemical compounds increases the risk of cancer, exposure to others may very well decrease the risk. So, in much the same way that vitamins and minerals prevent vitamin deficiency diseases, doctors and nutritionists are looking at ways in which some compounds may help prevent cancer. This new field is called *chemoprevention*.

Nutritionists and food scientists already know, for example, that certain vegetables contain compounds that may reduce the risk of cancer, and most of us are aware that colon cancer is less likely to develop in persons who maintain a high intake of dietary fiber. Similarly, some current studies illustrate roughly a 50 percent reduction in cancer risk among individuals consuming larger than average quantities of fruits and vegetables. The growing weight of such studies prompted the National Cancer Institute to launch a "Five a Day" educational program in July of 1992, urging Americans to eat five or more servings of fruits and vegetables every day. But thousands of compounds found in the diet have yet to be fully described, let alone studied carefully to discover their complete role in human health and nutrition. We can only hope that future study will reveal dietary elements that will protect us from specific cancers.*

One compound recently described as a chemopreventative and currently under intense scrutiny is quercetin. Quercetin (which also displays strong antioxidant properties) is a flavinoid derivative, one of a class of compounds that has very potent and easily demonstrated anticancer effects. As early as 1988 scientists showed that quercetin strongly inhibits the growth of a particular human cancer associated with squamous cells (both in the test tube and in patients). Subsequent work confirmed that quercetin acts to block a common oncogene.

Most of the compounds reputed to be chemoprotective share the chemical property of being antioxidants. According to recent work at the University of California in San Francisco, antioxidant properties also help to explain the effectiveness of dietary constituents and drugs used to reduce cholesterol. Is there a possible commonality among agents that have chemoprevention effectiveness and LDL cholesterol–lowering properties? This subject awaits further research, but 1993 reports confirm the presence of several antioxidants in wine, including resveratrol, which has a strong positive effect on blood lipids.

TO YOUR HEALTH!

Because quercetin is found in red wines but not in beer or spirits, there is at least theoretical reason to believe that the effect of wine on cancer risk is quite different from that of other alcoholic beverages. In fact, the few existing studies that examine the relative cancer risk due to wine, beer, and spirits suggest an increased risk for beer and spirits drinkers but not for wine drinkers, although results are not conclusive. Though quercetin occurs in much higher concentration in onions, broccoli, garlic, and several other foods, it shows no cancer-inhibiting activity in its native form and becomes active only when exposed to fermentation (as in wine) or when subject to bacterial action, as in the colon. Hence, other dietary sources of quercetin show anticarcinogenic action only when delivered to the large intestine, whereas quercetin in wine has anticancer activity from the moment it is put in the bottle at the winery. Because the majority of gastrointestinal cancers occur closer to the mouth than the colon, this is likely to be an important point in favor of wine. Furthermore, squamous cell carcinoma, in which quercetin is a particularly effective counteragent, is the type seen in 90 percent of esophageal cancers.

Although the low concentration of quercetin in wine causes most scientists to doubt whether it could have any positive anticarcinogenic effect, this issue will be decided in future research. But the existence of a potent anticarcinogen in wine, even in small quantities, illustrates once again the "special" character of wine in the diet as compared with other alcoholic beverages. It provides a plausible physiological basis for an anticancer effect of wine, an effect given further support by recent evidence that mice given wine as their drinking fluid had a suppression of induced cancer.

RESULTS

In trying to assess the relative risk of cancer from various sources, we need to recognize that many elements in the diet can cause cancer. By contrast, the evidence linking alcohol separately to the development of any sort of cancer shows up only for very heavy alcohol intake or is based upon very shaky and disputed data, without an animal model or a plausible mechanism. We can find no consistent evidence anywhere specifically linking wine drinking to any sort of increased risk for cancer.

So, although the same cannot be stated unequivocally for spirits or for beer, scientific opinion confirms that drinking wine in light, regular quantities does not cause any known form of cancer. In fact, even in very heavy wine drinking, any increased risk of cancer appears to be related to the concomitant use of some other cancer-causing substance or exposure, such as tobacco. Moreover, there is theoretical reason to believe that drinking wine can help *protect* against the development of cancer, and this possibility has been reinforced by epidemiological studies.

According to estimates accepted by the World Health Organization, cancer causes 20 percent of all deaths in North America and Europe, yet no more than 3 percent of that total is possibly due to heavy alcohol consumption. This means that if alcohol use were eliminated altogether, the maximum possible reduction in total mortality could be no more than 0.6 percent. By contrast, cardiovascular disease causes about 50 percent of total deaths, with light, regular wine drinkers enjoying about a 40 percent reduction in their risk of this disease. If alcohol were eliminated entirely, the possible small decrease in total deaths because of reduced cancer risk would be accompanied by an enormous, if not easily calculated, increase in deaths due to cardiovascular disease.

We believe that the light, regular wine drinker interested in low cancer risk should ignore any warning signs in the wine section of the supermarket* but be

*California law requires warning signs in wine shops to alert the public that drinking alcohol may cause cancer. If the federal government estimates that alcohol consumption may cause no more than 3 percent of cancer deaths (and some experts insist that even these cases of fatal cancer require the presence of tobacco exposure or some other initiator) while dietary factors cause at least ten times as many, what are the implications for butcher shops, supermarket meat departments, and steak houses, not to mention products like milk and butter, which contain large amounts of animal fats? Should these also carry warning of increased cancer risk?

sure that, in addition to a bottle of wine, the grocery cart contains such foods as carrots, onions, garlic, broccoli, cauliflower, cabbage, beans, squash, sweet potatoes, spinach, mangoes, cantaloupe, and other fruits, vegetables, and fiber-rich foods.

Chapter 5

Women and Wine

To read recent media reports, one would think that women should never drink a single glass of wine. It increases their risk of breast cancer, imperils unborn children and nursing infants, and puts women at increased risk of alcoholism as compared with men. In fact, some critics do maintain that women of childbearing age should abstain totally from wine consumption.

Just how realistic are these warnings? To answer this question we need to first determine wine's relative impact upon women and men and consider some important physiological differences between the sexes. It is true that there are many medical and health-related differences between women and men in addition to obvious sexual considerations;* beyond this, women and men show a variety of metabolic, anatomical, and physiological differences, some of which importantly influence the impact of wine drinking. As doctors we are especially aware and concerned about these distinctions. Good medical practice always depends upon the doctor's understanding of specific characteristics of the patient, and gender is merely the most obvious.

DRINKING AND DRUNKENNESS

One of the most important factors influencing the effects of a given quantity of alcohol on the body is the percentage of body weight due to fat versus water. Alcohol absorbed by the body from the stomach spreads throughout the total body water but is not distributed to fatty tissue. This is an important consideration for women because, except at the extremes of conditioning, women's bodies generally contain a greater percentage of total body fat than do men's, regardless of the "shapeliness" or physical fitness of the individual. Because fatty tissue contains no water, women have a smaller total body water content as a percentage of body weight (about 50 percent) than do men (about 60 percent).

*Beyond medical problems relating specifically to the reproductive tract and sexual organs, women suffer more from autoimmune diseases such as lupus, rheumatoid arthritis, and multiple sclerosis.

TO YOUR HEALTH!

Hence, a woman has a lot less water in her body than a male of the same weight. The fact that women also tend to be smaller than men accentuates the overall effect. If we take the example of an average woman weighing 130 pounds and a man weighing 180 pounds, the woman would have approximately thirty quarts of water in her body whereas the man would carry approximately forty-nine quarts—more than one and a half times as much total body water!

Therefore, if the man and the woman in the example both drank the same quantity of alcohol at the same rate, the woman would experience a much higher blood alcohol concentration. In fact, if this couple were drinking together and he consumed enough to produce a blood alcohol concentration of 0.075 percent (below any state's legal threshold of presumed impairment), his companion would have a blood level of about 0.12 percent or greater—well above the legal limit and clearly in the range that normally impairs motor performance, cognition, and judgment.

Although evidence is sketchy, it would appear that women also have less alcohol dehydrogenase (the enzyme that degrades alcohol before it can be absorbed into the bloodstream) in their stomachs. With less of this enzyme, women would absorb a greater percentage of alcohol consumed than men would.

Some women already know through experience that they do not seem to be able to drink as much as male companions. But the fact that a safe amount of drinking for an average man can cause an average woman to be very drunk is an important practical point that we all need to be aware of.

WOMEN AND WINE

Many public officials and some doctors will tell you that "a drink, is a drink, is a drink." We even see this message proclaimed in public service spots on television and radio. In fact, the official stance of the Bureau of Alcohol, Tobacco, and Firearms and various law enforcement and other governmental agencies includes this teaching. Despite this widespread public dogma, and as hard as it may be to believe, research demonstrates that *drinking different beverages with the same amount of alcohol* can result in quite different blood alcohol concentrations.

For example, drinking wine or beer causes a significantly lower blood alcohol level than consuming the *same amount of alcohol* by way of high-proof spirits under the same circumstances. This is true for both men and women, and drinking without food magnifies this difference, as much as 250 percent in some studies.

This is another important fact for women because it means they can decrease their potential for getting intoxicated by being sure that they drink only wine or beer, that they drink only with food, and that they drink approximately half as much as their male companion (assuming he is also drinking safely). For practical purposes, an average woman can have two glasses of table wine with food at a meal without risking intoxication.*

If the entire amount of alcohol in two 4-ounce glasses of wine (12.5 percent ethanol) were dumped directly into the bloodstream and caused to distribute immediately so that no metabolism could occur, the maximum theoretical

Among the most difficult and divisive issues that women face are the various controversies surrounding their biological role as mothers or potential mothers. Women who choose to become mothers owe the unborn child an enormous responsibility from the moment of conception. Mothers may adversely affect the health of the fetus through a variety of lifestyle choices and nutritional decisions. Even after birth, maternal lifestyle choices and nutritional decisions continue to influence the child's growth and development.

Some of these risks are obvious and relatively well defined: For example, health care workers in the United States estimate that tens of thousands of cocaine-addicted babies are born every year as a result of maternal crack cocaine abuse. Also, mothers who smoke during pregnancy expose their babies to various health risks, including an increased risk of sudden infant death syndrome (SIDS.) Even mothers who smoke after the baby is born increase the risk of SIDS in their offspring.

---

blood level that a 130-pound woman could achieve would be less than 0.08 percent (76 milligrams per deciliter). Practically speaking, even if gulped down as quickly as possible, alcohol absorption occurs slowly and incompletely, especially if taken with food. Metabolism begins in the stomach before any alcohol absorption and continues in the liver as alcohol absorption proceeds, resulting in a peak blood alcohol level below 0.04 percent, dramatically lower than the calculated value, and well below a level that one would consider intoxicating.

Another lifestyle choice and related risk (though much less well defined) relates to the question of drinking during pregnancy and fetal alcohol syndrome (FAS). There are some who feel that if drinking a little wine early in pregnancy can have a deleterious effect upon the fetus, a woman of child-bearing age who is not practicing a foolproof method of birth control should not have any amount of alcohol at all. But is it possible that a woman who is a light, regular wine drinker may expose her unborn child to a toxic dose of alcohol even before she knows she is pregnant? Let's look at what is known about FAS.

Twenty years ago, no one had ever heard of fetal alcohol syndrome. In 1973, the British journal *Lancet* published a paper that first coined the term, labeling a specific group of abnormalities in babies born after continuous exposure to heavy alcohol levels in utero. These babies all had low birth weights, together with a peculiar flattening and malformation of the face, often with an abnormally small head. They grew poorly after birth, and they showed various kinds of central nervous system deficiencies, with long-term mental retardation.

Although these birth abnormalities had been previously reported, many researchers did not initially believe they were caused by consumption of alcohol. Previously, scientists and doctors had taught that alcohol had no effect upon fetal development (as recently as 1983, prominent obstetricians in Ireland argued that fetal alcohol syndrome did not exist in that country, which is well known for heavy drinking of spirits). Eventually, however, the 1973 paper galvanized the scientific and medical communities.

Today FAS is a well-recognized syndrome, and the tragedy of its effects on infants cannot be overstated. Happily, it continues to be the subject of a great deal of research in the United States and abroad.

But just what are the risks of FAS? The National Research Council reported in 1989 that alcoholic beverages are the most important known human chemical teratogens (agents that cause birth defects), a statement that has been widely and repeatedly quoted. However, controversy continues even now over just how many babies are born each year with FAS and to what extent other variables contribute.

For example, the total incidence of fetal malformations of all kinds in the U.S. population is in the range of 80 per 1,000 live births, the vast majority of which are caused by unknown factors. And, in 1991 leading researchers at Wayne State University's Fetal Alcohol Research Center acknowledged that their earlier estimate of the incidence of FAS in the United States was six times too high; they currently estimate that roughly 3 out of every 10,000 babies may show evidence of FAS. Thus, of every 800 malformed babies born in the United States, only three-tenths to four-tenths of 1 percent are the result of maternal alcohol abuse. While some authorities assert that alcohol is the leading known cause of birth defects, the defects in 796 out of every 800 malformed babies are caused by something other than alcohol. Furthermore, research tells us that all these babies are born to mothers who habitually abuse alcohol *through-out* their pregnancies. (The majority of these cases come from poverty-stricken urban areas and Indian reservations.)*

Some recently published studies show a tendency for slightly reduced birth weight, slightly reduced motor performance at twelve months, and slightly reduced IQ at age seven among children whose mothers report that they drank as little as two drinks daily. This news has given rise to the idea that more subtle and limited forms of fetal damage may be connected to smaller amounts of maternal alcohol consumption, and some physicians even feel that any alcohol consumed during pregnancy can have a harmful influence on the developing fetus. Thus the term *possible fetal alcohol effect*, or simply *fetal alcohol effect* (FAE), has been coined. However, when we look at the evidence for FAE at the low doses of alcohol associated with light, regular wine drinking, we discover very weak and inconsistent findings. In fact, we cannot find an animal model for such a low dose effect, and human experience seems against it: Too many Italian and French geniuses sprang from wine-drinking mothers.

Animal experiments *do* confirm the existence of a vulnerable period and define a threshold for detecting a fetal alcohol effect. The vulnerable period, during which expo-

---

Because of the enormously inflated risk of FAS among Native Americans living on reservations (as high as 3 to 5 per 100) and among poverty-stricken urban minority populations, the authors at Wayne State University believe there may be some overreporting of FAS; other writers believe doctors underreport FAS.

sure to alcohol can cause damage to the embryo, varies, but exposure during the earliest phases of gestation causes no effect. If damage is to occur, the exposure must take place at a point later than that corresponding to about four weeks in humans. As for the threshold, it is clear that long-term low-level alcohol exposure causes no measurable effect, but relatively brief exposure to high levels at certain critical times does cause injury.

Although these results were obtained with animals, human studies mirror the results and reveal no difference in the birth weight or development of newborns from mothers who drank moderately during pregnancy as opposed to mothers who drank rarely or abstained. In fact, one report studied babies born to alcoholic women who had behavioral intervention during their pregnancies, leading to a reduction of their heavy drinking. Babies whose mothers drank heavily only during the first trimester had no central nervous system deficit, and there were no FAS babies. Mothers who drank heavily only during the first two trimesters gave birth to babies who showed a detectable delay in verbal development and a small risk of FAS. Children who were exposed to heavy drinking throughout pregnancy scored less well on measures of mental and language development and carried a higher risk of FAS. This little-publicized information demonstrates the importance of intervention in alcoholic mothers. If we can identify high-risk mothers early in their pregnancies and get them to reduce their drinking, their babies can be spared the tragedy of FAS.

There is an important lesson to be drawn from all this information. Throughout the literature of toxicology one can find examples of thresholds below which a given substance is quite safe and above which it is dangerous. Similarly, one might even see protective effects at low doses of otherwise toxic chemicals.* In fact, some physicians believe that low doses of alcohol may actually improve the probability for healthy pregnancies and healthy offspring.

Finally, in large studies, babies born to nonalcoholic, well-nourished, affluent or middle-class mothers do not show any measurable risk of fetal alcohol syndrome or fetal alcohol effect. By contrast, babies born to Native American or ghetto-dwelling women who drink heavily have the highest incidence of FAS/FAE. Although all babies born with FAS are the product of alcoholic mothers, even in the highest risk populations, at least 97 percent of babies in the highest risk groups are free of detectable fetal alcohol effect at birth (and some workers estimate the figure to be much higher).

To summarize our findings regarding FAS: Although it is not a trivial problem, early workers dramatically overstated its prevalence, and alcohol abuse accounts for no more than 0.4 percent of all fetal malformations. Despite two decades of intensive research, the mechanism by which high-dose alcohol exerts its effect upon the develop-

---

*A 1990 report in the Proceedings of the National Academy of Sciences of the USA stated that "almost everything we eat contains carcinogens, mutagens, and teratogens." The authors also repeat an axiomatic truth of toxicology, "The first rule of toxicology is that all chemicals are 'toxic chemicals'; it is the dose that makes the poison."

TO YOUR HEALTH!

ing fetus remains a mystery. Fetal alcohol syndrome occurs only in the offspring of heavy drinking, alcoholic mothers, and is especially related to binge drinking (at least five drinks on one occasion). It occurs most frequently in impoverished minority populations, particularly among Native Americans.

Also, heavy smoking and poor nutrition both separately increase the likelihood of FAS, as do use of other drugs, such as cocaine and marijuana.

BREAST-FEEDING

Although there is great variation in mothers' milk (depending upon her diet), doctors universally believe that breast-feeding provides the best possible nutrition for newborns. Breast-feeding also conveys such positive emotional-psychological effects as enhanced mother-infant bonding, reduces the overall risk for infection and allergic problems in the infant, and even possibly reduces the risk of breast or ovarian cancer in the mother. In light of these benefits, the obvious question for light, regular wine drinkers is whether or not it is safe for mothers to continue moderate drinking while breast-feeding. Could the exposure to alcohol in the breast-feeding infant cause a delay in mental development, motor coordination, or language development? Or could it show up years later as a tendency toward alcoholism?

Unfortunately, the research that has been done to date does not answer these questions directly. We do know that virtually all the dietary elements found in the mother's blood get passed to her breast milk, and alcohol appears in the mother's milk in approximately the same concentration as in the mother's blood. A baby who takes a full meal from the breast of a mother with a blood alcohol level of 0.12 (very drunk) can achieve a blood level of less than 0.01, but this (according to the Royal College of Physicians) is probably not significant.

On the other hand, we know that women who drink heavily expose their babies to other risks that are more readily quantifiable. For example, heavy drinkers are commonly heavy cigarette smokers, and we know that exposure to secondhand smoke poses a major health risk for children, including an increased risk for sudden infant death syndrome. This harmful exposure occurs whether the mother breastfeeds or not. Smoking mothers who breast-feed their babies also expose them to nicotine in the breast milk.

One study of twelve nursing mothers reported that babies who suckled shortly after the mother consumed the equivalent alcohol of a single glass of wine did not feed as well and slept more after feeding, but such effects are not restricted to alcohol: Women who follow their doctor's advice and exercise in the postpartum period will find that their baby may refuse to nurse after vigorous exercise; lactic acid in the milk makes it taste bad and persists for as long as 90 minutes. Another article reported a study of 400 babies and concluded that when measured at one year of age, babies whose mothers drank alcohol while nursing scored as well in a mental development test but slightly less well in a motor development test when compared with the scores of babies whose mothers did not drink while breast-feeding. Still, these findings are limited, and most doctors do not suggest giving up healthy drinking while nursing. In fact, an editorial accompanying the study of twelve mothers reviewed various findings of alcohol in relation to breast-feeding (including the study of 400 babies) and concluded that there is no reason to forbid mothers from light drinking during lactation, but that doctors should remind mothers of the fact that all drugs they take will pass into the breast milk.

It is also worth pointing out that many doctors (and the La Leche League) advise a glass of wine or other alcoholic beverage as an aid to relaxation for women who have difficulty initiating the flow of breast milk and maintaining it in sufficient quantities. Their feeling is that the benefits of helping mothers to breast-feed successfully clearly outweigh any risk posed by a small amount of alcohol in breast milk.

Finally, we might look to traditional cultures for some guidance in this area. Mediterranean cultures, for example, report a low incidence of problems associated with alcohol consumption, yet Italian women continue their usual habit of healthy drinking during the time they are nursing, as do mothers in Greece, Spain, and on the island of Crete.

WOMEN AND ALCOHOLISM

For thousands of years, men and women have enjoyed fermented alcoholic beverages. Literally throughout the historical record of civilization, positive references to wine abound, from Paul's biblical admonition to Timothy that he should "take a little wine for thy stomach's sake" to Louis Pasteur's remark that "a meal without wine is like a day without sunshine."

Many cultures have taken a different view when it came to women and wine, however. Ancient Rome, for example, prohibited women from drinking, afraid that they would be unable to control their sexual drive if allowed to drink wine. In the New World, excluding women from saloons and other drinking establishments continued well into this century.

Today we know that women are less likely to be abusive drinkers than are men: Most estimates report the incidence of alcoholism among women who drink as less than 5 percent, as opposed to the male incidence of more than 10 percent. The fact that light-to-moderate-drinking women tend to prefer wine may have something to do with this; women alcoholics, by contrast, generally prefer high-proof spirits.

Alcoholism in women, however, tends to be a much more rapidly progressive disease and tends to lead to more serious health problems than in men. For example, women may take only five years to progress to severe alcoholism, whereas the natural history for men may extend to twenty years. Also, women alcoholics have a much higher mortality risk than do male alcoholics.

For many years scientists believed men inherited genes that either would protect or predispose them to alcoholism, while women's tendency toward alcoholism depended much more strongly upon environmental and social factors. Very recent research has cleared up this question, however, and supports a much stronger genetic influence for women, probably identical to that for men. For both women and men one thing is certain: No matter how strong the genetic link, no one is a "born" alcoholic, and no one is genetically impervious to the risk of alcohol addiction. Today's research on problem drinking in general implicates genetic, social, relational, and environmental factors in developing alcoholism.

RESULTS

History, as well as the bulk of medical research, teaches us that the vast majority of women can safely and confidently drink wine from relative youth into old age without becoming problem drinkers or causing harm to their offspring. As long as she is drinking wine in a light, regular fashion, a young mother need not worry any more about the possible toxic effects of wine upon her unborn baby, or the infant at her breast, than about any other part of her diet. In fact, many other elements in the diet and environment as well as many other lifestyle choices constitute much stronger risks for injury and illness in women and their babies than any potential risk from light, regular wine drinking.

Women who enjoy light, regular wine drinking should evaluate any alleged risk of that habit in light of the readily demonstrated health benefits associated with this level of consumption. As shown in the cardiovascular chapter, women who enjoy light, regular wine consumption achieve up to a 40 percent reduction in mortality due to heart attacks, by far the leading cause of death among all women in the United States.

Consequently, we believe any woman who has shown herself to be a stable light, regular wine drinker, should be allowed to continue that habit without regard to whether she is pregnant or nursing a newborn baby.

Chapter 6

Wine and Mental Ability

The complexity of the human spirit has challenged thoughtful individuals since the beginning of history. From mythology and religion to philosophy and neurochemistry, we have tried to understand the mind. Today, we blend many disciplines, including psychology and neurobiology, with a growing emphasis on intracellular chemistry, to best understand mental function. Even this perspective will inevitably continue to evolve as we learn more and more about the brain's near infinite complexity. And because of the diffuseness of the concept, the diversity of functions, and the extraordinary range of influences that can play upon the mind, measuring the impact of any single influence is extremely difficult. The task becomes nearly impossible when you consider that influences operate at varying degrees of overtness, sometimes all at once and sometimes independently.

As a result, our knowledge about the impact of moderate wine drinking on the human mind tends to fall into four categories: First, "real-life" observations—these are not highly valued by scientists, because personal biases play too big a role. Second, laboratory situations in which at least some variables can be controlled and measured (this method has limitations as well: Our tools for measuring fall far short of perfection, and isolating wine drinking from its usual social context may change the psychic impact tremendously). Third, long-term studies of large population groups; and fourth, extrapolations from extreme cases. Here researchers take disease and impairment information gathered on alcoholics and others who have consumed toxic levels of alcohol and arbitrarily ascribe lesser effects to light, regular drinkers. This latter approach has no validity whatsoever in our view, yet it remains a common approach among the antialcohol bureaucracy. As we have stressed repeatedly, the effect of vast numbers of biologically active substances changes qualitatively with changing doses. (Attributing a destructive mental impact to light, regular wine consumption simply because megadoses clearly cause deleterious effects would be akin to saying that insulin at therapeutic levels must cause brain damage because insulin overdoses cause brain death.)

TO YOUR HEALTH!

Practically speaking, how many glasses of wine can one have before risking demonstrable impairment of intellect or behavior? The answer to this question varies with the individual's sex, weight, drinking experience, fatigue, emotional state, health, and the amount of food in his or her stomach. Also, adding complexity to the intellectual or behavioral test lowers the amount of alcohol needed to distort it.

Most of us are familiar with the charts used by law enforcement officers to predict illegal levels of alcohol in drivers. The chart reproduced here (Table C) comes from the California Department of Motor Vehicles and reflects the strictest standard in the country. In addition to California, five states (Oregon, Utah, North Carolina, Vermont, and Maine) currently use the intoxicated driver standard of 0.08 milligrams per 100 cubic centimeters of blood; the remaining forty-four states use the higher 0.10 level.*

If we want to understand this chart and interpret it correctly, it is important to know how it was derived. Those who construct such charts try to assure a 95 percent level of safety, meaning that fewer than five individuals in a hundred will exceed the 0.08 blood level after drinking the given number of drinks on an empty stomach. As you can see, a 130-pound woman will not exceed the 0.08 standard

*For simplicity's sake, charts such as this one equate the amount of alcohol in a 4-ounce glass of wine to that in a 12-ounce beer, or 1.25 ounces of 80-proof whiskey. The table does not reflect the reality that the body absorbs alcohol from wine and beer more slowly than from distilled beverages, or that wine is much more likely to be consumed with food.

TABLE C
Guide to Blood Alcohol Concentration

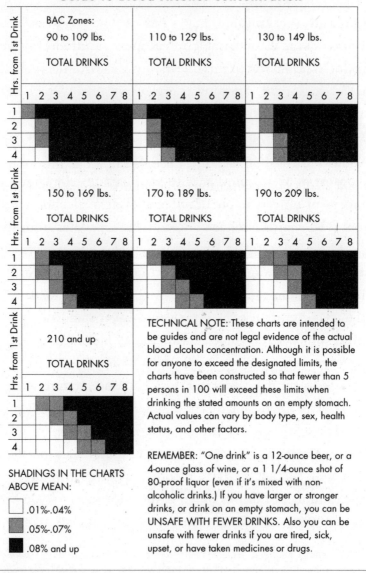

BAC Zones:

90 to 109 lbs. TOTAL DRINKS

110 to 129 lbs. TOTAL DRINKS

130 to 149 lbs. TOTAL DRINKS

150 to 169 lbs. TOTAL DRINKS

170 to 189 lbs. TOTAL DRINKS

190 to 209 lbs. TOTAL DRINKS

210 and up TOTAL DRINKS

(left vertical axis: Hrs. from 1st Drink)

TECHNICAL NOTE: These charts are intended to be guides and are not legal evidence of the actual blood alcohol concentration. Although it is possible for anyone to exceed the designated limits, the charts have been constructed so that fewer than 5 persons in 100 will exceed these limits when drinking the stated amounts on an empty stomach. Actual values can vary by body type, sex, health status, and other factors.

REMEMBER: "One drink" is a 12-ounce beer, or a 4-ounce glass of wine, or a 1 1/4-ounce shot of 80-proof liquor (even if it's mixed with non-alcoholic drinks.) If you have larger or stronger drinks, or drink on an empty stomach, you can be UNSAFE WITH FEWER DRINKS. Also you can be unsafe with fewer drinks if you are tired, sick, upset, or have taken medicines or drugs.

SHADINGS IN THE CHARTS ABOVE MEAN:

☐ .01%-.04%

▨ .05%-.07%

■ .08% and up

TO YOUR HEALTH!

unless she has at least three drinks in an hour or less, and a 210-pound man will be "safe" unless he has four or more drinks in an hour or less.

Nevertheless, driving performance, as well as other complex skills, depends upon a series of brain, motor, and sensory functions, each occurring in a timely and accurate fashion. Drivers must integrate these functions in a way that will assure smooth and competent behavior—safe driving. Studies clearly show that most people cannot do this with a blood alcohol concentration (BAC) of 0.10 or greater. However, though too much alcohol will impair anyone's performance, the effect is not strictly linear, and the precise pattern of impairment may vary considerably from one person to the next. Of course, substantial differences in driving ability exist even among sober drivers, and some evidence suggests that those with more limited skills to begin with are more likely to show impairment with smaller amounts of alcohol. One study even found that "variability among individuals in their responses to alcohol is far greater than any average effect." And though most individuals exhibited impaired performance at 0.10 BAC, a few individuals actually improved their performances. Another study reported similar results: Alcohol in low doses did not adversely affect the driver's ability to pay attention to two possible directions of motion. In fact, some observers' judgments of direction of motion became *more precise* rather than less. Finally, as the BAC falls below 0.10 and especially below 0.05, the effect on driving-related skills becomes less and less predictable, and more and more dependent on the individual.

WINE AND MENTAL ABILITY

As a practical matter, what we have defined as light, regular wine drinking—a single glass of wine for the average woman, one or two for men—presents little or no driving hazard, especially if the person is an experienced driver and/or the wine is consumed with meals. However, novice drivers, or those impaired by fatigue, illness, or disability—should never drive after drinking alcohol.

ANXIETY

Anxiety is a diffuse emotion, closely related to fear, that is experienced by everyone and perhaps best described as a feeling of unrest, apprehension, and even dread. Although it can be problematic, it also has true survival value in promoting arousal, vigilance, and coping strategies. Of course, most people become adept at treating anxiety in their own lives through nonchemical means. However, when anxiety becomes severe and/or persistent, many try alleviating their distress with various drugs. In fact, anxiety-relieving medications consistently top the list of "most popular" prescription drugs—and have done so for forty years. In any given year, 12 to 15 percent of the adult population in the United States will take such medications.

Though most people consume wine primarily for social and cultural reasons rather than for medicinal ones, physicians in the past traditionally prescribed a glass or two of beer or wine as treatment for anxiety or insomnia. Physicians generally believed that such doses lacked side effects and produced relaxation rather than intoxication, especially when taken with food or in the company of family or "responsible" friends.

In the nineteenth century, however, the growing pharmaceutical industry began developing an ever-evolving series of "miracle drugs" for treating anxiety. As a result, physicians favored a sequence of substances that could be put strictly under physician control and therefore presumably be less likely than alcohol to be abused or misused. Since then a continuing series of drugs—everything from bromide salts to barbiturates to Valium and Xanax—have been touted as more effective against anxiety than anything previously known while simultaneously being nonaddicting and free from side effects. Yet each has had problems and side effects, including addiction.

Unfortunately, relatively few studies (meeting contemporary standards) have examined wine's impact on anxiety. One 1991 study revealed that low-dose Valium and alcohol produced similar effects on subjective feelings in healthy young men, although the Valium resulted in "significantly more impairment than did ethanol on measures of memory, body sway, and the evaluation of the passage of time." A 1992 publication by the National Institute of Alcohol Abuse and Alcoholism (NIAAA) reviewed the available literature and suggested "that lower levels of alcohol consumption can reduce stress; promote conviviality and pleasant and carefree feelings; and decrease tension, anxiety and self-consciousness."

WINE AND MENTAL ABILITY

Should people who are anxious use wine or other alcoholic beverages to self-treat anxiety then? Ultimately, the answer means making a personal decision based on cultural values: Some groups find drinking alcoholic beverages for these purposes to be morally repugnant; others believe that alcohol-containing beverages provide a traditional and culturally satisfying way to reduce tension. On a practical and medical level, wine clearly fulfills a tension-relieving function and has been a favored treatment throughout the ages; and, at a light, regular level of consumption, the side effects of wine compare favorably with medications commonly prescribed for anxiety reduction.

THINKING ABILITY

Our ability to think distinguishes human beings from all other forms of life. Human thought encompasses an enormous range, from perception and distinction to computation, organization, and memory, to analysis, judgment, and reflection, among other processes. Although we know that intoxication at sufficiently high doses will affect all these processes, can we also say simply that high doses produce major impairment and low doses produce lower levels of impairment? Do we need to wonder about the implications for light, regular drinkers, that is, do they develop lesser degrees of impairment?

Most of the evidence here suggests the answer is no. Even the NIAAA, which refuses to use the term *responsible drinking*, declared in 1989 that data linking social drinking and cognitive impairment remains "inconclusive." The *British Medical Journal* reviewed the existing research in 1984 and reached the same conclusion: "we still have no good evidence to suggest that we need to revise the safe daily drinking limits of 60 grams ethanol for men [four to six glasses of wine] and 30 grams for women [two to three glasses]."

One authoritative overview commented that "low alcohol doses have been found to improve certain types of cognitive performance. Included here are problem-solving and short-term memory." But the single most authoritative review and critique of the literature concluded that the "findings are variable and seldom reproducible. There is no consistent evidence to support any of the causality hypotheses [that would suggest an adverse impact of social drinking on cognitive ability]."

DEPRESSION AND SUICIDE

Depression encompasses a spectrum of moods ranging from isolated symptoms to full-blown disease. Everyone experiences symptoms of depression during a lifetime. Feeling low or unhappy on occasion is simply a part of life, especially in response to events involving loss, disappointment, or failure of some kind. Depression *as a disease* occurs much less commonly but has a substantially more serious impact. Depression causes significant suffering and disability, and its most lethal consequence, suicide, causes up to 25,000 deaths in the United States yearly.

At any given time, perhaps 5 to 20 percent of the population will report having symptoms of depression. Such symptoms tend to be most common among people who have objective reasons for feeling unhappy, especially those who are physically ill, who have suffered a significant personal loss (e.g., due to death or divorce), financial problems, or other disappointment. Depression tends to be most common among people for whom life is hardest, including people from dysfunctional families, the elderly, people with chronic diseases, widows and widowers, the disabled, the unemployed, the institutionalized, and alcoholics.

Alcoholics, of course, tend to be people with substantial numbers of family and personal problems even before they begin to drink; and heavy-drinking alcoholics customarily develop numerous additional problems, including problems related to employment, relationships, physical illnesses, finances, and the law. Under these circumstances, no one should be surprised that alcoholics commonly report being depressed.

Alcoholics also appear to be predisposed to more serious depressions, including the lethal risk of suicide. One recent study suggests that up to 25 percent of suicides in the United States are associated with alcoholism. Heavy drinking not only increases the likelihood of a suicide attempt but may also contribute to the outcome, especially in suicide by drug overdose, where it can magnify the lethal nature of some commonly used drugs.

However, scientists do not know how much depression in alcoholics stems from problems with the external world, how much is due to the effect of alcohol itself, and how much should be attributed to other neurochemical variables caused by poor eating habits, sleep disruption, illicit drug abuse, and other factors. Each probably plays a part, with the degree of influence varying from person to person.

And though it is true that depressed alcoholics tend to become less depressed once they have achieved abstinence, no one knows how much improvement stems from pharmacologic actions of alcohol and how much may be related to simultaneously changing social variables. For example, as alcoholics become abstinent, their employment opportunities increase, their financial status improves, and so on.

The question remains, then, whether alcohol, as a chemical acting upon the brain, instigates depression. First, alcohol is classified as a central nervous system depressant, meaning that, in common with various other drugs (including benzodiazepines such as Valium) alcohol suppresses certain functions in the brain. For example, the apparent stimulation that social drinkers enjoy comes from a suppression of mechanisms involved in inhibition and social restraint. But does suppression lead to depression? The answer is no: Suppressing nerve function will not lead inevitably to a mood depression.

There is much confusion about this issue, even at times among health professionals, and most of it stems from the terminology used. Scientists use the phrase *central nervous system depressant* to refer to a chemical that suppresses the transmission of neuroelectrical impulses, not to imply an effect on mood. In fact, depression as a mood may have nothing to do with suppressed nerve transmission. "Central nervous system depression" and depressed mood are two entirely separate and distinct phenomena. In fact, although suppression of some brain functions may lead to depression, suppression of others may lead to exhilaration.

An enormous amount of research has examined the relationship between alcohol and depressed mood, but little of it has had to do with light, regular social drinking, especially of wine. So, though persistent heavy drinking correlates with strong symptoms of depression, no credible evidence suggests that light, regular consumption of wine causes depression.

What about light, regular wine drinking when a person is already depressed? Will it make that person's depression worse? Here the answer becomes more complicated and probably depends upon the context in which the drinking takes place. Alcohol, when consumed by a depressed person drinking alone, may add to the level of depression; when consumed as part of pleasant and supportive social interaction, the opposite appears to be the case, and the depression lightens.

A series of studies in several geriatric facilities, conducted from the mid-1960s onward, sheds more light on this issue. Researchers gave residents the opportunity to drink a glass or two of wine in daily social gatherings. The residents, men and women in their seventies, carried histories of being loners in the institutions. Some functioned "normally," and some were disoriented, with evidence of significant brain disease. In almost all cases, wine drinking produced dramatic changes for the better. Ward atmosphere improved significantly, with more lively communication and more general enjoyment. Fewer residents needed heavy tranquilizers or needed to be restrained. Even incontinence declined substantially.

The remarkable success of these early studies led to wine socialization programs at geriatric facilities around the country. By the early 1970s, other studies reported the same phenomenon. At a Chicago-area church-sponsored geriatric residence, the clearest findings were a three-to-one reduction in depressive symptoms among wine drinkers. Not one of these studies noted adverse effects.

A mid-1970s study fit the same pattern: increased morale, decreased worrying, more restful sleep, and no adverse effects. More recent studies among independently living adults in their sixties, seventies, and eighties who began drinking a glass or two of wine each evening also supported the earlier conclusions. Though not universal, positive changes in mood and morale were reported by the average participant.

However, the more severe the depression, the more careful one needs to be in consuming any alcoholic beverage. If depression reaches suicidal proportions, the risk level escalates, and alcohol should certainly be avoided.

RESULTS

In the average person, light, regular wine consumption has no adverse effect on mental health, including on that person's emotional tone and ability to think clearly, especially if he or she has good health and consumes wine with food. To the contrary, the bulk of the evidence suggests that light, regular wine drinking helps lighten the anxiety of everyday life and ease depressive symptoms when taken as part of social interaction.

Whether a person *should* drink wine for these purposes remains an individual decision, one that in our culture depends heavily on religious and cultural considerations. But from a strictly medical viewpoint, wine taken in the contexts discussed here remains a reasonable option for the vast majority who do not have any specific condition or vulnerability that would argue against use of alcoholic beverages.

Chapter 7

Contaminants and Additives in Wine

Although food contamination is as old as food, only recently have we been able to measure it in the minute quantities we now take for granted. As our methods of technical analysis become ever more refined and as our ability to find contaminants shifts from the parts-per-thousand level to the parts-per-million and parts-per-billion level of precision, we find contamination everywhere. We could argue, in fact, that our ability to detect contamination now far outstrips our ability to understand what the figures mean for human health.

LEAD AS A CONTAMINANT

In August 1991, the federal government released figures showing that many wines sold in the United States contained lead in quantities far above the amount permitted in drinking water. Although domestic wines had far lower levels than imports, the lead content for both jumped dramatically when the liquid was poured over the lips of bottles sealed with lead foil capsules. This information, made public under pressure from a group of food and nutrition advocates, left the public in a quandary: What did it all mean? The impact for many was to make wine seem a dangerous, disease-causing beverage.

Emphasizing the potential danger, an FDA spokesman said the agency would immediately propose a ban on lead foil capsules, explaining further that "although the lead levels found do not pose an immediate threat to consumers, we at FDA are concerned with long-term exposure." He said that the agency would also consider establishing maximum permissible levels for lead in wine.

To understand what was behind the FDA's decision, we must know a little about the issue of food contaminants generally, why they remain a continuing problem for virtually all prepared foods (and many "natural" ones as well), and see just how the question of wine and lead fits in with total mortality figures.

Lead seems to become a problem to human beings in direct proportion to its usefulness. Because it is durable, corrosion resistant, and highly malleable, it has been favored for making pipes as far back as Mesopotamia, and many older homes throughout the world still have lead plumbing. In Roman times, vintners added lead to wine, to keep it from spoiling while contributing a pleasant flavor. Although many drinkers subsequently suffered colic (described in the ancient Roman medical literature) it was not until the seventeenth century that lead was determined to be the cause.

The main effects of acute lead poisoning occur in the stomach. Symptoms include severe cramping or colic, nausea, vomiting, circulatory collapse, and even death in extreme cases. If lead is ingested in smaller amounts, chronically over a prolonged period of time, it affects the blood (resulting in anemia), and the nervous system, where both the brain and peripheral nerves experience damage.

Unfortunately, the body absorbs lead fairly easily, and, if the amount absorbed exceeds certain levels, the body suffers.* Scientists argue about the precise levels at which harm occurs, but everyone agrees that children are much more vulnerable to ill effects than are adults, and the younger the child, the greater the vulnerability.

Although adults also take in lead from food, thanks to governmental regulation, such sources as lead plumbing, lead solder, and lead glazes on dishware represent an ever

*Unlike other metals, lead serves no known function within the human body, even in trace amounts, and physicians generally presume that we can survive very well without lead.

smaller risk to our population. For example, currently only 3 percent of food cans produced in the United States have lead solder, whereas the figure was closer to 90 percent as recently as the 1970s. Nevertheless, some "background" lead in the soil and water will clearly be with us far into the future, because decades of leaded gasoline use have contributed over 7 million tons to our environment.

Currently, food products that have the highest levels of lead are those that are the most acidic, especially citrus fruits and juices, foods preserved in vinegar, tomato and apple sauce, brewed coffee, and alcoholic beverages such as beer and wine. Condiments also tend to be high, as do seafood and grain. Of course, storage containers that have substantial amounts of lead, such as lead-crystal decanters and lead-glazed ceramic pottery and dinnerware, significantly raise the levels of lead found in the foods they hold.

It is worth examining just how much lead can be found in these other products, especially as they compare with the lead content of wine. (In the table that follows, all levels are in parts per billion.)

A quick glance at the table reveals that many common foodstuffs, consumed by children as well as adults, contain substantially higher lead concentrations than bottled wine. Two of the highest, tomatoes and spinach, average three to seventeen times the levels found in wine. Why, then, did the topic of lead and wine grab all the headlines, instead of "tomato sauce and lead" or "spinach and lead"? There seems to be no ready answer available, but the media attention and political reaction to this issue are a matter of record.

TO YOUR HEALTH!

FOOD ITEM	MEAN LEAD CONCENTRATION	MAXIMUM LEAD CONCENTRATION
Domestic table wine	41 PPB	521 PPB
Imported table wine	94	673
Tuna (canned in oil)	167	570
Pork and beans (canned)	105	530
Peaches (canned in syrup)	181	440
Fruit cocktail (canned)	176	410
Pears (canned)	126	280
Spinach (canned)	422	1,650
Sauerkraut (canned)	270	930
Tomato sauce (canned)	164	980
Tomatoes (canned)	710	8,000
Mushrooms (canned)	196	480

Adapted from data from the Bureau of Alcohol, Tobacco, and Firearms and Gunderson, Ellis. For full citations, see bibliography for this chapter.

As mentioned earlier, the lead level increases substantially if a lead capsule seals the bottle*and the lead acetate deposits, which sometimes accumulate at the top of the bottle, are not wiped away with a cloth before the wine is poured. Fortunately, most wine drinkers always wipe away

*The lead foil capsules on wine bottles (actually a sheet of lead sandwiched between two sheets of tin) were all phased out on California wine by early 1992 (and are in the process of being phased out elsewhere), to be replaced by 100 percent tin foils or by aluminum, paper, or plastic components. Recently, many states—beginning with Connecticut, Iowa, Maine, New York, Rhode Island, and Wisconsin—passed legislation prohibiting the use of lead (and some other metals) in packaging materials generally. For wine bottles, the

such deposits, because lead salts on a bottle rim look like dirt. However, when 432 bottles were tested without wiping the lead deposits away, an initial mean level of 80 PPB escalated to 145 PPB after the wine was poured over the lip of the bottle. (As we can see from the table, this figure is still below that of the mean lead contents for canned mushrooms, sauerkraut, etc.). In imported wines, though, the mean decanted lead level was 195, and the figure reached well over 1,000 in a few decanted bottles from Algeria, Chile, Cyprus, Spain, and France.

Just what do all the PPB figures mean? Reviewing the past forty years of world literature on the topic, we found that for adults the minute levels found in wine and other commercially available foods—even where lead levels far exceed the EPA standard—have absolutely no relevance to clinically detectable disease. Though we came across a couple of dozen instances of lead poisoning traceable to wine, all but one involved homemade wines prepared and/or stored in lead-lined or lead-glazed vessels. The single instance of lead poisoning traceable to commercially sold wine was reported in France in 1968 and concerned two individuals who had consumed wine that had been transported in bulk in lead-plated containers.

Some might argue that lead poisoning from wine has probably been underdiagnosed and underreported, and we

---

foil historically served to keep rats from chewing corks in long-cellared bottles, as well as helping keep oxygen out of the bottle in days before corks and bottle size were completely standardized. Currently, lead foil serves a primarily decorative function.

TO YOUR HEALTH!

would agree that this is likely. However, the same could be said for virtually all other kinds of poisoning related to food and drink. Most doctors, ourselves included, treat minor and transient clinical problems on the basis of clinical symptoms only. We do not order batteries of expensive tests for lead or various obscure chemicals or pathogens, as long as the patient gets better. Therefore, though we may well have missed diseases caused by lead in wine, we are just as likely to have missed those from lead in spinach or from contaminants in water, fruit juice, and milk.

The fact remains that diseases related to lead in wine (or in other foods) have been reported only rarely, and these rare instances should be contrasted with far more common instances of disease and even death from other contaminants.*

The world's greatest overall public health hazard is impure or biologically contaminated water, a problem encountered universally in third world or developing countries, causing an estimated 12,000 deaths per day due to infectious diarrhea.

"Advanced" or industrialized countries receive only partial immunity. The Environmental Protection Agency estimates that industry, agriculture, and municipal sewer systems together discharge some 200 billion gallons of

*Another measure of wine's minute role in toxic exposures can be seen from poison control center statistics. In one recent year (1989), seventy participating centers reported over 1.5 million poisonings. The most common sources of toxins were cleaning substances (160,652) and analgesics (160,591). By contrast, lead poisoning accounted for 2,005 reports, with but one death. Nowhere was there evidence that any of these poisonings were wine related—or food related, for that matter.

CONTAMINANTS AND ADDITIVES IN WINE

sewage daily into U.S. water supplies. One EPA report listed 253 identifiable organic chemicals commonly found in U.S. drinking water, with such compounds as acetone and chloroform being found in all municipal systems tested, from Grand Forks, North Dakota, to Lawrence, Massachusetts.

In 1993, almost 300,000 people served by the Milwaukee water system were suspected of being infected with a diarrhea-causing organism, due to inadequate processing at the treatment plant. A 1990 report described the contamination of Tucson, Arizona, drinking water with trichlorethylene, which researchers believed to be statistically linked with congenital heart disease in several hundred children.

No one can guarantee you that any food you eat is free of contamination.

A recent article in the *Journal of Food Protection* reported that an average of 12.6 million cases of food-borne disease occur each year, with 84 percent having microbiological causes. Most cases involve relatively mild, transient "food poisoning," but even so, diseases such as botulism, hepatitis, listeriosis, salmonellosis, and the like account for five hundred deaths a year.

In 1988 the U.S. Food and Drug Administration reported a study of foods purchased at retail outlets around the country, each of which was examined for contamination by selected pesticides, industrial chemicals, and elements. An average of sixty-four contaminants were found in each market basket of 234 foods. The most contaminated foods were

baking potatoes, with twenty-seven chemical residues and 115
fresh/frozen spinach, with twenty-six.

In 1992, a U.S. government investigation revealed that
as much as 20 percent of our seafood shows evidence of microbiological deterioration or chemical contamination. Because fish and shellfish often live in contaminated water,
they constitute the largest single food source of dietary
toxic chemicals and pesticides, as well as being the largest
single source of food-borne illnesses.

Even milk, that cornerstone of childhood nutrition,
seems fraught with hazard. A 1989 article reported out-
breaks of bacterial contamination of pasteurized milk and
cheese that caused one hundred deaths from meningitis,
abortion, and perinatal septicemia. The *Journal of the
American Medical Association* reported an Illinois epidemic with over 16,000 culture-confirmed cases of salmo-
nella in two brands of pasteurized milk affecting over
150,000 persons, making this the largest outbreak of salmonellosis ever identified in the United States.

It is clear that, in light of all this, public concern about
wine and lead seems vastly out of proportion to the evidence for its danger. If recent journal articles are any indica-
tion, the average American consumes far more lead from
water and canned fruit juices than from wine, and probably
runs the greatest risk of disease from milk or fish. Similarly, the FDA's decision in late 1991 to advise all health
professionals "to warn pregnant and nursing mothers that
wine containing even low levels of lead may pose a hazard

CONTAMINANTS AND ADDITIVES IN WINE

to the fetus or nursing infant" seems arbitrary, discrimina-
tory, and reflective of an antiwine bias. Why not impose
these same warnings for lead in tuna fish, fruit cocktail,
fruit juice, or spinach, among many other food categories?
Why not warnings about potential bacterial contamination
of milk, a problem that has clearly killed more people than
lead in commercially sold wine, or a warning on all water
faucets about chemical contamination of municipal water
supplies, a problem that appears to have caused dramatically more congenital abnormalities? One can only wonder
what caused the agency to select out wine from all other
consumables.

SULFITES AND ADDITIVES

In 1985, federal agencies became increasingly concerned
about sulfite preservatives added to various foods. By Sep-
tember of that year, the government logged fifteen "confirmed deaths associated with sulfites." One case that got
particular press attention occurred in Dallas, Texas, on July
11, when a thirty-three-year-old man drank some German
wine and had a sudden, fatal reaction. The apparent cause
was sulfite (in the wine), a compound the deceased had
been advised to avoid because it might trigger his asthma.

Subsequent government hearings led to important regulatory decisions: The FDA prohibited the use of sulfites on
raw fruits and vegetables—an action directed primarily at
salad bars—and most (but not all) sulfite-containing foods
and drugs had to be labeled. The Bureau of Alcohol,

Tobacco, and Firearms (BATF), which regulates wine, soon followed suit and required that all wine containing more than ten parts per million of sulfites also needed to carry a warning label.

What Are Sulfites?

At the time these reports began to surface in the news, most Americans had never heard of sulfites. Even today many of us may wonder what they are and why anyone would use them in food and drink. More important, exactly how dangerous are foods that contain sulfites?

The term *sulfites* covers a variety of chemical compounds, including sulfur dioxide, sodium sulfite, sodium bisulfite, sodium metabisulfite, potassium bisulfite, and potassium metabisulfite. Added in carefully controlled concentrations, these compounds prevent food spoilage from bacteria and fungi and prolong shelf life by preventing browning or discoloration of various foods. (They perform this same function in medications, so numerous pharmaceuticals also contain sulfites.) Hundreds of everyday foods contain sulfites, although consumers cannot always tell from the product label. These include fresh, frozen, canned, or dried fruits and vegetable products (including jams, juices, and syrups), shellfish, baked goods, soups, snack foods, condiments, and salad dressings and sauces, as well as beer and wine.

The sulfite used in winemaking is sulfur dioxide, which vintners add to the amount produced naturally during fermentation. Although many vintners refrain from adding sulfites to wine, nature makes it impossible to exclude the compound entirely from the fermentation process.

Sulfur dioxide's use in wine production goes back centuries. Early winemakers burned elemental sulfur, causing it to combine with oxygen. The resulting fumes disinfected barrels and other implements involved in the winemaking process. Its antioxidant properties also prevent excess oxygen from combining with certain constituents in wine to produce discoloration and deterioration in taste. However, the amount must be strictly limited, because excessive amounts produce unpleasant odors that spoil the taste and aroma.

Sulfites, Allergies, and Wine

For the vast majority of consumers, sulfites are virtually undetectable and absolutely safe. Unfortunately, for about 5 percent of asthmatics (who themselves constitute about 5 percent of the population), as well as for other unusually sensitive people, sulfites can pose a significant risk, ranging from relatively minor allergic reactions to fatal effects.

Food allergies are frustratingly individual: Most people are not allergic to any given substance, and those who are allergic may not be equally allergic all the time. Also, a concentration that may be tolerable on one occasion may be intolerable on another, and the biological response on a given day can range from minor and irritating to lethal.

Some people have "allergic reactions" after eating a given food raw or only partially cooked but have no reaction after eating the food completely cooked. Others require certain foods in certain combinations before they have reactions. Others with moderate sensitivity have reactions only when consuming extraordinarily large amounts of a given food. And though some individuals develop food allergies as they grow older, others seem to outgrow their allergies.

Estimates vary widely concerning the prevalence of food allergies. Two out of five Americans believe they are "allergic" to some food, but an American Medical Association article estimated the true figure to be 1 to 2 percent of the adult population. Part of the reason for this discrepancy has to do with the definition of allergy. Physicians distinguish between foods that make people sick because the foods contain toxins, foods that some consumers find to be disagreeable or upsetting to the stomach, and foods that cause a systemic immunologic reaction—a true allergy.

Though we do not know the exact numbers of specific food allergies, 90 percent are probably caused by the "big four": milk, eggs, nuts, and fish. As for food additives, those that produce true allergic reactions tend to be preservatives and antioxidants such as sulfites. However, other additives, such as various coloring agents (coal tar dyes), preservatives (nitrates and nitrites), and flavoring agents (monosodium glutamate and aspartame, or NutraSweet®) also produce reactions—including asthmatic attacks—in susceptible people.

Most allergic responses are minor and involve skin reactions such as a rash, diffuse itching, and swelling. Asthma is relatively more rare but also significantly more troublesome; anaphylaxis*—the most serious allergic reaction of all—remains very rare. Naturally, these serious and potentially lethal reactions also arouse the most concern.

Against this background, how does wine fare in comparison with other foods? No doubt exists that some people have allergic reactions to wine, but wine's contribution to food-related allergies remains relatively trivial. The few additives allowed by law include yeast culture, some sugars, acids and alcohols derived from other grapes, the sulfur dioxide mentioned earlier, and sorbic acid (which serves to limit yeast proliferation in sweet wines). Although many other compounds can theoretically end up in wine (and every other agricultural product) including herbicides, pesticides, fungicides, and fertilizer components, regular testing by wineries and regulatory agencies almost never turns up even a trace. As a practical matter, though dozens of additives are legal and safe according to the FDA and BATF, few actually find their way into wine. Most commercial wineries use sulfur dioxide but no other additives.

However, adverse reactions to wine occasionally crop up in the medical literature. As with reports on all food-related allergies, only some of them stand up to scrutiny. One report examined eleven asthmatic patients who thought they had severe reactions to alcoholic beverages. Only six showed significant problems when tested in the laboratory, and of the five people who thought themselves allergic to wine, only

*Anaphylaxis is an acute, sometimes fatal, multisystem immunologic response. In the most severe cases, cardiovascular collapse and breathing cessation may be immediate and resistant to all efforts at treatment.

three had any measurable response. Though a smattering of similar articles exist, the number remains remarkably low, considering the billion or so individuals who drink alcoholic beverages around the world each year.

In forty years of medical literature, during which hundreds and hundreds of millions of people consumed wine on countless occasions, only one death occurred in which anaphylactic reaction to wine alone was the probable factor. This is the death in the thirty-three-year-old Texas man that was so influential in leading to the 1986 sulfite-labeling decisions.

What about other deaths that were supposedly related to sulfites? The FDA's Center for Food Safety and Applied Nutrition (CFSAN) reviewed "27 deaths temporally associated with sulfiting agents," examining autopsy records, where available, medical records, clinical and dietary histories, and toxicology studies. Despite all the scare headlines about sulfites that appeared in the mid-1980s, not a single death among those scrutinized by CFSAN can be attributed to sulfites conclusively. In virtually every instance, other allergies or other factors might be involved: CFSAN concluded that thirteen were either not related to sulfites or unlikely to be related or that there was no clear evidence to decide one way or the other. Of the remaining deaths, nine were "strong possibilities" for an association with sulfites, but of these, three had consumed sulfited potatoes, two had eaten sulfited lettuce and guacamole, and others had sulfited vegetables or lemon juice. In only two cases was wine consumed. A forty-four-year-old woman drank white wine—

but also ate from a sulfited salad bar and ate a pizza that may have contained sulfited ingredients. The second wine drinker is the same man from Texas we discussed previously.

Since 1982, at least nine fatal allergic reactions to nuts and seeds reached the medical literature, in addition to dozens of near-fatal events. We uncovered at least two fatal anaphylactic reactions to fish and shellfish and scores of near-fatal events due to various fruits, vegetables, milk products, and grains. In the United States each year, four hundred to eight hundred people die from allergic reactions unrelated to wine.

RESULTS

The problem of toxic elements—whether contaminants or additives—is often a real one, and it should concern all of us. However, so too should we be concerned with the facts. If there is a potential for taking in toxins, whether through food or by way of such environmental hazards as lead paint, we should all do our best to protect ourselves and our children; but if there is no danger, we should not be asked to alter our lifestyles needlessly—there are plenty of good reasons to make changes.

The facts about food contamination are that, though it sometimes stems from the processes of food preparation and packaging, more often it comes from the chemical and bacterial contamination in our environment (due to our inability to adequately treat our industrial, agricultural, and human waste). Lead poisoning in particular should be seen for what it is: primarily an environmental hazard for children and secondarily an industrial hazard for adults in certain occupations. Despite the sensationalist headlines, lead poisoning does not present a real hazard for adults with regard to any commercially prepared food. More specifically, *absolutely no evidence exists to suggest that lead poisoning poses a significant problem in drinking commercial wine.*

Similarly, we must be able to separate the facts from the scares when it comes to additives in food. Though wine and the vast majority of other packaged foods we purchase all contain additives and these additives (as well as some natural constituents in wine) do cause infrequent allergic reactions in susceptible people, 99.75 percent of the population has no allergy to wine. More importantly, allergic reactions to wine are far less common than similar reactions to nuts, milk, fish, and eggs.

Thus, if a single death were sufficient reason for warning labels on all wine bottles, there should be significantly larger labels on foods that contain peanuts, processed nut meat, and perhaps even peanut oil, to mention only one example. It seems, instead, that regulators subject wine to a different, more harshly demanding allergic standard than they do other foods. From a medical point of view, this discrepancy makes no sense: When it comes to additives and allergic reactions, wine remains far safer than many other foods we take for granted and for which no warning labels are required.

Chapter 8

Alcoholism, Abuse, and the Perception of Risk

THE RISK OF ABUSE

Of all the health risks associated with alcohol, none arouses more passion than abuse. Some contend that, for specific vulnerable individuals, any taste of alcohol will start the drinker down the path of alcoholism and lead to multiple drug abuse and a ruined life. Statistics commonly quoted by antialcohol forces suggest that as many as 10 percent of drinkers will suffer significant problems related to alcohol consumption sometime during their lifetime. On the other hand, the alcohol beverage industries maintain that the vast majority of people drink in a "normal," controlled, moderate fashion and will suffer no significant adverse consequences as a result of their consumption.

Yet even determining what alcoholism is and who can be said to abuse alcohol is no simple task. Though ordinary citizens may feel reasonably sure they know what constitutes abuse, scientists have much more difficulty coming up with a consensus. The thinking about this issue continues to evolve. For example, doctors first officially labeled alcoholism a disease in the 1950s. Before that, most people regarded alcoholism merely as evidence of moral weakness.

The disease concept of alcoholism has resulted in more compassionate treatment of the alcoholic, and it has provided a veritable windfall for those in the health professions involved with alcoholism research, prevention, and treatment. An outspoken coalition of national and local lobbying groups—organizations ranging from professional associations to volunteer coalitions, with both religious and lay sponsorship—vigorously promote the disease concept. But more recent definitions broaden the concept, separating out alcoholism, alcohol-related organic mental disorders, alcohol abuse, and alcohol dependence. Today, most experts define alcoholism in terms of a collection of biological, psychological, social, and cultural variables, each of which can be plotted along a continuum. Of course, the precise cutoff point of each—where one decides to differentiate between nonalcoholism and alcoholism—tends to be highly arbitrary and subject to personal rather than medical values.

Unfortunately, no currently accepted definition relies on the quantity or frequency with which alcohol is consumed, and none requires "excessive" drinking, however defined. Alcoholism professionals can apply the problem-drinker label to the one-drink-a-month man, as well as to the ten-drinks-a-day woman. The concepts of alcoholism and alcohol abuse are now so diffusely defined that practically anyone who consumes alcohol, no matter how rarely or how small the amount, could be labeled a "problem drinker." There are even "hard-liners" in the alcoholism movement who view any use of alcohol whatsoever as equivalent to abuse.

Alas, the people who formulate these definitions have a vested interest in seeing the problem defined as broadly as possible, afflicting as many people as possible. In a sense, it is like putting the fox in charge of the hen house, except that we have also let the fox define hens so broadly that the hen population includes ducks, rabbits, squirrels, pigeons, and virtually all other critters to the fox's liking.

Screening Tests

Because the definitions of alcoholism, alcohol abuse, and alcohol dependence are themselves so fuzzy, no one should be surprised that the devices used to screen large population groups for the prevalence of these conditions exhibit little precision. Consequently, the results, that is, "What percent of our population suffers from these conditions?" range across a considerable spectrum.

Though there are dozens of screening instruments for detecting "problem drinkers," the most popular is probably the CAGE questionnaire. The CAGE's wide use stems from its brevity and ease of administration. Its supporters claim it to be up to 97 percent sensitive (meaning it can identify 97 percent of problem drinkers in any study group) and 94 percent specific (meaning that, of "problem drinkers" identified by the survey, 94 percent of them actually will be "problem drinkers," and only 6 percent will be falsely labeled). The test consists of only four items. Two or more positive answers identify the problem drinker:

1. Have you ever felt you should cut down on your drinking?
2. Have people annoyed you by criticizing your drinking?
3. Have you ever felt bad or guilty about your drinking?
4. Have you ever had a drink first thing in the morning to steady your nerves or get rid of a hangover? *

Though supporters enthuse about the CAGE, the test suffers from several major flaws. First, values of the persons in the responder's immediate vicinity mightily influence answers to the first three questions. Therefore, a woman who had no objective evidence of alcohol-related problems might respond yes to questions one, two, and three even if her only alcohol consumption were a glass of champagne at

*The first article documenting the CAGE Questionnaire was printed in The American Journal of Psychiatry 131 (1974): 1121–23. Permission to reprint the questions here has been granted by the American Journal of Psychiatry.

TO YOUR HEALTH!

a wedding once or twice a year, when she was surrounded and criticized by vocal teetotalers. The "problem" in such a circumstance may have far less to do with the drinker than with the disparity in cultural values between the drinker and those in her immediate social circle.

Furthermore, feelings of guilt are not necessarily the best gauge of an abuse problem. If women of average or below average weight worry about being overweight—which is precisely what 75 percent of "normal" American women do—most physicians would say that they have anxiety problems, not weight problems. But according to the CAGE, if an average or infrequent drinker worries about that drinking, it is not evidence of an anxiety problem or societal pressures but of an alcohol problem.

Finally, to put into perspective the significance of answering yes to the first three questions, try substituting words or phrases such as "eating candy," "frequent golfing," "watching television," or "working long hours" for "drinking." Though candy lovers, dedicated golfers, TV aficionados, and hard workers might indeed have some problems juggling these activities with other priorities and pressures, few would say that responding positively to the first three questions automatically meant that such problems warranted the label of disease.

Despite these flaws, surveys based on questionnaires such as the CAGE determine most of the estimates of alcoholism and alcohol abuse in this country. It is not surprising, then, that such instruments find alcohol problems in large numbers of those surveyed.

ALCOHOLISM, ABUSE, AND THE PERCEPTION OF RISK

The "Core" of Alcohol Abuse

When alcoholism becomes fully developed, it envelops the whole of a person's life and body, producing a clinical picture achingly familiar to nurses and physicians everywhere: cirrhosis of the liver, brain malfunction, including memory loss and confusion, withdrawal seizures, pancreatitis, bleeding from the stomach, anemia, yellow jaundice, and even toxic psychoses, as well as other less dramatic but nonetheless debilitating problems. For someone approaching such an advanced clinical stage, alcoholism truly constitutes a chronic, progressive disease that inevitably will be fatal if treatment fails. Though the vast majority of individuals who have alcohol-related problems (however defined) never become so profoundly ill, no one doubts alcoholism's potential destructive impact, including grief not only for the afflicted but also for family, friends, and innocent parties as well.

Yet no matter how broadly some people seek to define "alcoholism" and "alcohol abuse," the most worrisome societal issues stem from a few core behavioral problems and some specific alcohol-generated diseases. Because it involves so many innocent people, perhaps the most tragic of these problems is drunk driving. How big is the problem, and to what degree does the light, regular wine drinker contribute?

In 1991, car crashes killed 41,462 individuals. Of that number, fewer than half were "alcohol-related events." Experts consider a fatal traffic accident to be alcohol-related if either a driver or nonoccupant has a detectable level of alcohol in the blood, no matter how low or how high the level. For example, if a man who has had one beer goes to sleep on a park bench and that bench is run into by an entirely sober driver and the sleeper is killed, the fatality qualifies as alcohol-related.

Despite the fact that 65 to 70 percent of Americans and 95 percent of adult male drivers consume alcohol, in 1991 almost 70 percent of all drivers involved in fatal accidents had blood alcohol levels of zero. Naturally, the innocent victim statistics tug most at our heartstrings, but, at the same time, we need to remember that more innocent victims die from non-alcohol-related traffic events than from alcohol-related events. In addition, "alcohol-related" accidents seldom involve only alcohol. For example, fatigue and sleep-related transportation accidents play a role in 30 to 40 percent of highway accidents, killing up to 10,000 people each year.

When measured in deaths per vehicle miles traveled, the trend gives us cause for cautious optimism. In 1966, with one trillion miles covered in this country, the fatality rate was 5.5 per 100 million vehicle miles. In 1990, with more than two trillion miles, the National Highway Traffic Safety Administration estimated the rate at 2.1, "the lowest recorded fatality rate in history." Thus, the highway death rate has dropped over 60 percent in 25 years. Obviously, safer vehicles, seat belts, air bags, and such have been a significant factor in the decline, but happily a smaller percentage of fatalities due to drunk driving is also partly responsible. From 1982 to 1988, the percentage of drivers who were legally drunk and involved in fatal accidents decreased from 30 percent to 24.6 percent.

Finally, a steady accumulation of studies confirms that the usual drunken driver drinks heavily as a matter of habit, regularly consuming five and more drinks per occasion, has a general disregard for traffic laws, and has a tendency toward high-risk behaviors in general. The phenomenon of fatal drunk driving stems from a very small portion of the alcohol-consuming population. And the light, regular drinker is involved in a minute portion of fatal accidents relative to the percentage of such individuals in the driving population.

Public drunkenness is another significant problem in this country. In 1989, police arrested more than 800,000 people for public drunkenness—5.7 percent of total arrests in the country. Violent offenders also commonly consume alcohol prior to their crime: Persons arrested for assault often have alcohol on board, and up to half of rape offenders drink at the time of their offense. Heavy drinking plays a significant role in falls, burns, homicides, domestic violence, other trauma, and a wide variety of antisocial behavior. But the association of violence with alcohol does not mean it is the cause. Many antisocial individuals have problems with substances other than alcohol, as well as a variety of psychological and interpersonal difficulties above and beyond their substance abuse, and no evidence exists to indicate that alcohol is a causal factor in violence at levels that characterize the light, regular drinker. We can find no studies that suggest light, regular wine drinking is involved in violent behavior.

TO YOUR HEALTH!

So, though the antialcohol community commonly regards alcohol as a "cause" of antisocial and violent behavior, alcohol use in and of itself is neither a necessary nor a sufficient explanation for undesirable activities. As long as 70 percent of our population consumes alcoholic beverages, 70 percent of people involved in any activity will tend to be drinkers, and 30 percent will tend to be abstainers. What is important is that occasional and light-to-moderate drinking are the norm in this country; heavy drinkers and abstainers remain the exception.

Risk Factors

Why is it that most people drink but only a small percentage become alcohol dependent? No matter how we define alcoholism and alcohol-related problems, or how we interpret the statistics, it is clear that not everyone is equally vulnerable to becoming an alcoholic or to having alcohol-related problems. Different cultural and ethnic groups, for example, vary enormously in their vulnerability. Jews, southern Italians, and Greeks rarely suffer from alcoholism, whereas northern Europeans and Native Americans tend to be much more vulnerable. Also, though per capita consumption of alcohol varies considerably from one country to another, the countries with the highest numbers are not necessarily the countries with the highest percentage of alcohol-related problems. Some cultures encourage responsible drinking habits; others foster less responsible drinking.

One major study, widely quoted and very influential, regards the most important predictors of alcoholism to be alcoholic parents, alcoholic ancestors, and cultural background. Future alcoholics, in other words, come from cultural groups that accept adult drunkenness while simultaneously not teaching children safe drinking practices.

Although the relationship seems to be complex, genetics clearly plays some role. Papers published in the past dozen years report studies of adopted children of alcoholics and nonalcoholics followed over time, and the results suggest that genes transmit some predisposition to alcoholism. The most widely accepted model postulates that genetics determines who has an addictive-type personality. Environment will then either foster and promote this tendency toward addiction or thwart it by way of positive and negative reinforcers.

Alcohol as a Gateway Drug

Antonia Novella, U.S. Surgeon General during the Bush administration, was a fierce opponent of alcoholic beverages and developed a special crusade against underage drinking. She pointed out that about half our teenagers have tasted alcoholic beverages and as many as 8 million consume alcohol on the average of one or more times a week.

Novella saw alcohol as a drug rather than as a desirable component of some foods and beverages. Under her leadership, the Public Health Service promoted the notion that alcohol use is equivalent to abuse and tried to direct the public's intense negative feelings about illicit drugs toward alcoholic beverages. She was alarmed that most teenagers take their first drink when they are thirteen and contended that alcohol use is often the first step on a pathway to multiple drug abuse.

Unfortunately, there was no recognition that the overwhelming majority of teenagers who are introduced to alcoholic beverages in a responsible way by their families go on to become responsible adult drinkers. For example, among religious Jews, all teenagers are considered to become adults at age thirteen and are expected to drink small glasses of wine in religious services with the adults. The alcoholism rate among Jews is among the lowest in the world. If wine is a "gateway drug," it clearly is not uniformly so.

Where Does Wine Fit In?
Though current estimates suggest that about 65 to 70 percent of Americans consume alcoholic beverages one or more times a year, nobody knows how precise that number is or what percentage drinks how much or how differing percentages behave while they are drinking. If you take the most dire statistics at face value, about one in ten drinkers (and thus one in fourteen Americans) risks becoming an alcohol abuser.

Yet looking at the statistics from another perspective, that means 90 percent of Americans who drink do so responsibly. In addition to this figure, virtually every available survey suggests that, among drinkers in general, wine consumers behave the most responsibly. The explanations are conjectural, but most authorities point to the fact that wine drinkers, in the United States, consume their beverage primarily with meals and/or as a part of family, social, or religious events. Surveys reveal that 75 percent of wine consumption takes place in home-based family settings; of these, four-fifths are in the consumer's home at mealtimes, particularly supper. These are settings that encourage responsible behavior.

If consumers do drink wine away from home, restaurants make up the next most common setting. The average intake is only a glass and a half, an amount highly unlikely to produce intoxication, interfere with judgment, or impair driving in an adult.

While as many as 42 percent of Americans drink wine, a 1990 study revealed that, of legally impaired drivers (with BACs of 0.10 or greater), only 3 percent were wine drinkers, and a 1988 report by the Department of Justice found only 2 percent of drunken driving arrests involved wine drinkers.

Thus, even though 90 percent of those who drink, drink responsibly, when it comes to wine, the figure approaches 98 percent. That means that about 2 or 3 percent of wine drinkers risk problems of abuse. We should not ignore this figure, but neither should we let it frighten us. How many things in life can we identify that are abused by fewer than 3 percent of users? The automobile? Sex? Our legal system? Television? And at what level do we let the acknowledged difficulties of a tiny minority determine health choices and public policy for the rest of us? Should our concerns about 3 percent of our number lead us to punitive restrictions on the other 97 percent? The truth turned around still remains the truth: What carries danger for the few can be beneficial and safe for the many.

WINE AND HEALTH: IS THE RISK WORTHWHILE?

In the preceding chapters, we examined the effects of moderate wine drinking on various parts of the body and in relation to specific social issues. We saw that wine has both positive and negative effects depending on the level of consumption. We also saw that wine shares these qualities, in varying degrees, with other foods and beverages—none is perfect. Anything powerful enough to provide benefit can also create harm. How the risk compares to the benefit depends upon individual health needs and choices and other dietary constituents. It can all be maddeningly diffuse and vague, but certain patterns do emerge.

As a beverage, wine has middling nutritional value. Such beverages as milk and orange juice clearly contain more nutrients. On the other hand, wine packs substantially more nutritional value than such beverages as coffee, tea, and soft drinks. With regard to the cardiovascular system, no other food or beverage reduces overall mortality or the incidence of heart attacks more than wine. Given that cardiovascular disease is overwhelmingly the nation's number one killer, this is a remarkable statistic. Still, certain people cannot drink wine because of palpitations or because their blood pressure becomes elevated. Light, regular wine consumption, though carrying substantial benefit for the heart, is by no means a perfect solution.

For the average person, light, regular wine consumption probably produces little impact on the gastrointestinal tract. Some with sensitive stomachs may find that wine produces gastritis in the same way that caffeine-containing beverages, acidic juices, and some spicy foods do; others may feel that wine aids in the digestion of fatty foods. Light, regular wine consumption has no demonstrable effect on the healthy liver or pancreas.

Compared to other common foods, wine *in the amounts advocated here* probably has little or no impact on conception, fetal development, pregnancy, delivery, or breast-feeding, but women who feel themselves particularly vulnerable or who feel burdened by taking even marginal risks may want to avoid it altogether while pregnant or breast-feeding. (However, the same women should exercise the same degree of caution with strenuous exercise or any food likely to be contaminated with organisms or potential toxins, particularly prepared foods, milk and cheese, fish, or municipal drinking water.)

When it comes to cancer, the Surgeon General says that people who consume alcoholic beverages heavily have a 2 to 3 percent increased risk of cancer, and this risk rises for cancers of the mouth and upper digestive tract with individuals who smoke. Most newer studies indicate that wine may have a protective effect against some cancers, but these relatively modest effects, pro and con, must be contrasted with the Surgeon General's estimate that animal fat increases the risk of cancer generally in the range of 35 percent.

With regard to human behavior, thought, and aptitude, research has yet to demonstrate any consistent adverse effect due to light, regular wine drinking. To the contrary, wine has a well-established beneficial effect on anxiety, and when consumed in a social setting can reduce the depression and even confusion related to social isolation. Although some studies suggest adverse effects on higher thinking and fine motor behavior, they are balanced by others that indicate salutary effects, and absolutely no evidence indicates long-term adverse effects on thinking in lifelong light, regular drinkers.

Another criticism of wine drinking is the potential for consuming various contaminants or additives. But studies on lead in wine and other foods reveal that numerous foods have higher lead levels. Moreover, intensive research failed to unearth a single modern example of any adult's getting lead poisoning from any commercially prepared food or beverage.

In terms of sulfites, additives, and allergic reactions, wine ranks very low on the risk scale. Allergic reactions to nut products, fish, fruit, eggs, and milk far outshadow the relatively infrequent problems associated with wine.

The single greatest risk associated with the light, regular consumption of any alcoholic beverage is that low-level consumption can escalate to abusive consumption, and with abusive levels comes the potential for a variety of well-recognized and undeniable problems: drunk driving, deterioration of functioning in family or on the job, legal and financial problems, not to mention major health problems. But what level of risk does the average wine drinker face? The answer depends on how one defines abuse and varies with certain genetic and social factors. For the United States as a whole, 7 to 12 percent of alcoholic beverage consumers risk becoming abusive drinkers. Wine drinkers are the least likely of all drinkers to have problems related to abuse, however. Surveys reveal that wine is the alcoholic beverage least likely to be consumed to the level of drunkenness, and that only 2 to 3 percent of people arrested for drunken driving report drinking wine.

First Benefit, Then Risk

All this begs the question, How can you measure the benefit of wine drinking and factor in the risk? We can get some readily understandable and practical guidance if we look at an example of one of wine's beneficial effects and compare it to other things that offer similar results: reducing the risk of heart attack.

According to a *New England Journal of Medicine* article that analyzed nearly two hundred studies for their impact on the prevention of heart attacks, the single most useful strategy (50 to 70 percent reduction of risk) requires stopping smoking. A variety of other interventions can reduce risk in the 40 to 50 percent range: reducing serum cholesterol, treating high blood pressure, maintaining a physically active lifestyle, maintaining ideal body weight, and consuming "mild-to-moderate" amounts of alcohol. Taking prophylactic doses of aspirin lowered risk in the 33 percent range.

The authors stopped short of recommending "mild-to-moderate" alcohol consumption, citing their concerns that low consumption might escalate to high consumption, saying "the difference between drinking small-to-moderate quantities of alcohol and drinking large amounts may mean the difference between preventing and causing disease."

Another study, published the following month in the *Annals of Internal Medicine*, came to the identical conclusion: After reporting a decade-long study of 11,688 men in which mortality from coronary artery disease declined significantly and in a linear fashion as men consumed two drinks or more per day, the authors nevertheless concluded that "alcohol consumption cannot be recommended because of the known adverse effects of excess alcohol use."

Unfortunately, these conclusions imply that alcohol consumption involves significant risk but that other interventions and strategies commonly recommended by physicians to decrease cardiovascular risk—from weight reduction to exercise to prophylactic aspirin—carry either zero or minimal risk. Such an implication is patently false. Given its dramatic protective effect against the nation's number one killer, light, regular wine consumption carries a relatively small risk *for most people.*

The Perception of Risk and Wine's Place
in Medical Therapeutics

Why do today's physicians commonly recommend weight loss, exercise, aspirin, and various other medicines to control cardiac risk factors but become wary and stern when discussing light, regular wine consumption, which has comparable cardiac benefits and no more risk?

It is likely that most physicians—being largely cautious and conservative people—have succumbed to current concepts of "political correctness" and have allowed contemporary social values and pressures to influence their medical thinking. And, because we are a nation obsessed with the dangers of substance abuse—understandably so—we have enormous difficulty in objectively weighing the risks and benefits of any substance that has the potential for abuse, however small that potential may be. Finally, and not the least of possible reasons, is that physicians have become so wary of litigation that avoiding political hot potatoes has become a priority for most.

Yet speaking only from a medical perspective, we now believe that light, regular wine consumption has clear health benefits for the majority of individuals concerned about their cardiac risk, and—again from a medical perspective—cardiac risk reduction should concern the majority of the population. Wine also has its health risks, particularly for that minority of individuals who are vulnerable to addictive or abusive behavior, but none of the strategies to reduce cardiovascular risk are danger free. In fact, all the other recommended strategies—quitting smoking, losing weight, exercising, or taking aspirin, blood pressure, or cholesterol-lowering medications—involve significant risks.

Still, different individuals will weigh those risks differently, and it is quite human to fear risk in activities you do not like and to minimize risk in activities you do like. No activity can be risk free, but danger, for all of us, is a matter of degree.

Our lives would become much easier if any given food, beverage, or activity were either clearly safe or clearly unsafe. Instead, we deal with varying degrees of risk mixed with varying degrees of benefit, and these risks and benefits vary in importance to different groups of individuals. A continuing flow of ever-evolving scientific information constantly presses us to reassess our own perceptions and judgments.

Consequently, we believe that when most reasonable people consider all the evidence, many will agree that light, regular wine consumption remains a sensible and relatively safe option for reducing cardiovascular risk, not to mention a safe component of an enjoyable lifestyle. We recommend it to most sensible adults on that basis.

Relative Risks

Throughout this book we have seen that smoking represents one of America's greatest health risks. Indeed, physicians generally agree that smoking-related conditions are the most common preventable causes of premature death today. Besides being directly responsible for over 100,000 deaths per year from heart disease, smoking accounts for considerable mortality from lung and other cancers, chronic lung disease, vascular disease, and other diseases as well.

But is quitting smoking without its own risks? Certainly not. For almost anyone, quitting carries a small risk of major adverse consequences and a moderate risk of temporary and minor but potentially very bothersome consequences. These are some of them:

- Each year, more than three out of four people who try to stop smoking will fail; they will experience the adverse emotional consequences that commonly accompany failure: depression, anxiety, lowered sense of self-worth, and the like.
- Whether successful or not, quitting almost always involves withdrawal symptoms—cravings, anxiety, restlessness, impatience, sadness, inability to concentrate, weight gain, bowel irregularity, sore gums, sore tongue, increased phlegm, and emotional irritability. The importance of these symptoms, and their consequences, varies considerably from person to person. (For example, a relatively placid person may find an increase in edginess and a shortened emotional fuse to be tolerable; a person who already has problems with a short temper or who works in a high-risk profession such as poiice work may find these symptoms much less acceptable.)
- One common method of fighting nicotine withdrawal is use of transdermal patches (although they have yet to be proven

effective in long-term studies). These come with a long list of warnings, some minor and some potentially serious: Allergic reactions occur in about 10 percent of users during six weeks of use; they should not be used in pregnancy or during nursing; users need to be particularly cautious if they have histories of cardiovascular disease, liver or kidney disease, peptic ulcers, hypertension, or hormonal problems; over a third of patch-wearers tend to have localized skin reactions. Finally, there is the possibility of carcinogenesis and impairment of future fertility, both of which are listed on the product warning label.

- For many people, the likelihood of weight gain presents another major obstacle to giving up smoking. According to one study, 10 percent of men and 13 percent of women gain as much as, or more than, twenty-eight pounds.
- Finally, numerous studies indicate that people with histories of major depression have much more difficulty stopping smoking than normal individuals, and that when such people attempt to stop smoking, they risk deepening their depressions, even adding to the risk of suicide.

What do these facts indicate? Simply that even *quitting* smoking involves risks. For the vast majority of people, the health risk remains small compared to the health benefits. But consider the case of a single mother supporting her children in a job for which appearance and a slim figure have undisputed importance. If this woman also has problems with depression and knows that she tends to become short-tempered with her kids, this might not be the best time in her life to try to give up smoking. And though the vast majority of physicians (including ourselves) recommend stopping smoking for those patients who still use tobacco, a sensitive physician would also temper those recommendations depending upon the circumstances involved. They should do so because they perceive that, for some people,

ALCOHOLISM, ABUSE, AND THE PERCEPTION OF RISK

the clear health benefit must be balanced by an awareness of risk.

Let's look at another example. There is very strong evidence to indicate that maintaining what doctors term "ideal body weight" will provide substantial protection against the risk of heart attack. But can individuals achieve and maintain ideal body weight without risk to health or well-being? Current research suggests yes for some people and no for others. In fact, weight loss creates a number of problems and potential health risks for many people:

- Because we are a country obsessed with food, on the one hand, and the numbers on the bathroom scale on the other, awareness of weight and body image pervades our culture. A 1992 survey, reported at the National Mental Health Association meeting, revealed 40 percent of youngsters in grades five through eight feel fat and want to lose weight.
- Repeated surveys demonstrate that three-fourths of women whose weights are clearly normal by medical standards feel themselves to be fat and wish to lose weight. The harvest in terms of guilt, anxiety, depression, distorted self-image, and frustration is common knowledge. Worse, our national obsession has generated an epidemic of eating disorders. Up to 10 percent of adolescent and college-aged women are afflicted with anorexia nervosa and bulimia.
- Recent evidence suggests that biological variables, especially genetics, have enormous impact in influencing body weight and shape. For those whose genes lead them to exceed "normal" weight, undergoing strict diets and strenuous exercise paradoxically may make them less rather than more healthy.
- Specific regimens, most notably the liquid diets, have been linked with gall bladder disease, headaches, nausea, dizziness, and even sudden death. Other diets carry risks of spe-

cific vitamin and mineral deficiencies. In general, dieting commonly causes irritability, impaired concentration, craving, anxiety, depression, guilt, and the like.

Obviously, though maintaining "ideal body weight" carries strong health benefits, dieting and trying to reach this ideal is not risk free and for some may be considerably more problematic than others.

Let's look at one more example of a health benefit with significant associated risks: physical activity, especially sports. Nowhere has the medical profession ignored the risks inherent in a prescription as much as it has when encouraging patients and the general public to participate in regular exercise.

Almost all physicians (including ourselves) regularly recommend exercise to our patients. We do so because we share a cultural bias in favor of physical activity and because good medical evidence exists that such activities can have both physical and psychological benefit. Likewise, the American Heart Association regards physical inactivity as a major risk factor for heart disease and recommends a wide variety of activities, including jogging, basketball, and other sports.

If asked, most physicians would say that participation in exercise involves minimal risk and that severe injury or death occurs rarely. However, injury and death do occur, and far more frequently than most of us would like to admit. In fact, thousands die sports-related deaths each year in this country, and millions sustain sports-related and exercise-related injuries that result in temporary and sometimes permanent disability. Let's look at some facts:

- A 1989 *New England Journal of Medicine* article reported that bicycling resulted in almost 600,000 emergency room visits and 1,300 deaths per year. Bicycling also accounted for 900,000 head injuries from 1984 to 1988, according to a 1991 article in the *Journal of the American Medical Association.*

- Another article, from a journal specializing in sports medicine, asserted that athletics account for 6,000 preventable head injury deaths and "literally millions" of less severe head injuries annually. Each year, football head injuries alone produce approximately 250,000 concussions and eight deaths.

- A British journal found that, of severe eye injuries requiring hospitalization, 42 percent occurred during sport or athletics; a similar American article estimated that sports account for nearly 25 percent of severe eye injuries.

- The *American Heart Journal* revealed that of the 17 million American joggers, 8,000 "have been killed by automobiles and over 100,000 injured" during a single year. Moreover, any physician who commonly treats runners can recite a litany of minor but nevertheless aggravating problems, including foot, ankle, hip, and back disorders, tendonitis and myalgias (muscle pains). Runners who pursue their sport along congested city streets commonly inhale high levels of ozone, sulfur dioxide, nitrogen dioxide, and carbon monoxide, sometimes causing symptomatic problems and sometimes permanent damage. As one lung specialist observed, "Guys jogging in place next to cars at a stoplight . . . might as well smoke a cigarette."

- The *American Heart Journal* also attributed approximately 25,000 sudden *cardiac* deaths to exercise and athletic activities. That is an incredible figure, meaning that 5,000 more people die *cardiac* deaths due to sport than die from alcohol-related traffic fatalities each year. This figure does not include *traumatic* deaths from sport, for example, the 1,300 people who die in bicycle accidents each year.

What does all this mean? Certainly we are not implying that sports or athletic activity should be discontinued, or that sporting equipment should carry warnings of the risk of death. Nor do we suggest that four-pack-a-day smokers give up the thought of quitting or that seriously obese persons abandon their attempts to reach a healthy body weight. Instead, we wish to remind readers that many pleasurable activities, even those with statistically significant health benefits, *also* involve risk.

The point is that most activities—sensible, light, regular exercise, for example, just like sensible, light, regular wine drinking—may involve some small health risks. As exercise becomes more vigorous, with higher impact activities, the risk of serious bodily harm increases substantially, much the same as with drinking alcoholic beverages! So, these risks should certainly be taken into account, because any individual's decision will rest upon personal values and how one applies the perceptions of relative risk and benefit to oneself. But, similarly, the relative benefit must also be taken into account, whether it is a healthier body maintained near the recommended ideal body weight or a healthier cardiovascular system from light, regular wine drinking.

Chapter 9

Teach Your Children

GUIDELINES FOR SOCIAL POLICY

For thousands of years, the vast majority of people around the world have enjoyed wine as a sensible part of a happy and healthy way of life. From the beginning, it has also been true that some individuals abused wine; but it has always been clear that at the root of the problems were those who abused, not the drink itself. Wine remains a highly desirable beverage for most of us, who continue to feel that problems experienced by the few should not mean the majority must do without.

In the past, too, concerned, sensible, well-intentioned people fought hard to balance the needs of the temperate majority with risks to the intemperate minority. In wine, as in life, we—like our ancestors—struggle to find the happy medium.

Today, we continue the struggle in a new language: We speak in terms of health rather than religion, morals, and character. Thus for the past quarter century, the single most powerful argument in favor of any given social policy has been "it would be good for the health of our people." Politicians and lobbyists use medicine and health to argue for or against issues as diverse as distributing condoms in schools, restructuring the workplace, and implementing organic farming techniques. Unfortunately, any argument that is applied so widely lends itself to misuse; partisans on both sides bolster their positions with fragments of research and convenient opinions from carefully selected health professionals. Extremely vocal groups now see health in evangelical terms, rather than in terms of personal medical decision making.

The result of so many health-related decisions influenced by so many diverse groups is an ever-growing umbrella of policy that tries to encompass the interests and values of all players. Unfortunately, it inevitably bends to pressures exerted by a few passionate voices tying their views to high-profile human interest stories. A good example is reports of accidents involving drunk drivers that arouse more attention and usually weigh more heavily in alcohol policy decisions than the far more common drinking of wine in quiet family gatherings. The loser in these conflicts is almost always the man or woman who lives within the rules, the person for whom extreme positions are neither relevant nor meaningful.

Typical of this new policy mentality was the 1987 national prohibition forbidding the purchase of alcoholic beverages by individuals under twenty-one, regardless of whether they are married, parents, or members of the armed services. Thus, the law prohibits a twenty-year-old Desert Storm veteran, responsible enough to earn his living carrying an assault weapon, from buying a bottle of wine or beer for himself or even champagne for a wedding or birthday.

The most fervent participants in public policy discussions about alcohol tend to be people who understandably feel their lives irrevocably damaged by alcohol abuse of one kind or another: former alcoholics, who now spend their time convincing the general public that what was disastrous for them, personally, will inevitably be disastrous for the many, and individuals with a family member killed by a drunk driver.

It is not surprising that the carnage perpetrated by drunk drivers has absorbed our nation's attention. In this century we have been slow to learn to deal with the challenge of drunkenness and the automobile (inebriates no longer injured only themselves by falling off a horse or stumbling on their walk home from the tavern, but command multi-ton machines capable of killing whole groups of innocent victims). In the last decade, however, deaths due to drunken driving decreased because we developed effective laws against it and enforced them vigorously. This seems to be the logical path: Drunk drivers are the problem, not drinking.

Whatever our newfound dilemmas about technology, wine remains what it has always been: a pleasant and healthful commodity that can and will be abused by a small but nonetheless significant minority of people who drink it. Yet light, regular wine drinking is not the same thing as alcohol abuse; and though use and abuse are not entirely separate, neither are they identical. Use and abuse range across a spectrum, with the precise dividing line varying from one person to another, depending on individual health and vulnerabilities. But some people find such complexity offensive. If wine in large amounts creates problems for a few, some prefer to argue that wine in any amount will be bad for the many.

Ironically, just the opposite is true. For most, light, regular wine drinking has only a strongly positive effect on cardiovascular health and overall longevity; otherwise, it remains overwhelmingly health-neutral. Compared to much on our menu—from milk to fish to peanuts to ordinary drinking water—wine stacks up remarkably well from a health standpoint.

Wine and Policy

Those are the facts about the effects of wine and how policy is made. We must now decide what we are going to do with them: We know that light, regular wine consumption has a healthful effect on the vast majority of the population—are we willing to use that information to actively promote a responsible drinking culture instead of a "Just say no" culture?

Unfortunately, antialcohol lobbies, the federal government, and even a portion of the medical literature all suggest that the public should be protected from the knowledge of wine's healthful qualities. As we have already mentioned, the government refuses to recognize the concept of healthful drinking, and alcohol regulatory agencies refuse to let wineries mention that their beverage has healthful qualities. Even competent medical scientists who do acknowledge wine's healthful contributions nonetheless balk at recommending wine to people who could benefit from it.

These observations lead us to an inescapable recommendation for setting new policy: We urge that future health policy efforts distinguish between use and abuse of legal and traditional beverages such as wine. In fact, we feel that there will not be a safe, responsible attitude toward drinking until all those who contribute to policy in this country recognize this fact.

The Scare of the Day

Most of the scientific information available to the average American comes from the popular press, and, understandably, it is usually presented in a way that they hope will grab our attention. The downside is that at times hype replaces fact. And rarely will someone ask on the public's behalf what such and such really means compared to what we thought last year or last decade, or what it means when compared to apparently conflicting research reports.

Of course, the public cannot expect to look to persons on either side of the issue for an objective critique. Business groups too often downplay risks and hazards associated with their products (though they run liability risks in doing so). Public interest groups, by contrast, gain money and funding by emphasizing hazards and run no liability risks in promoting fear and anxiety. Regrettably, neither group feels any special responsibility for the welfare of the average consumer; indeed, no group, publication, or institution carries a mandate to help the public sort out the latest "health scare of the day" in a balanced and useful fashion.

We need some mechanism to help us put this ever-increasing avalanche of information into useful perspective. Most of us understand the impossibility of a totally risk-free environment, but we need authoritative help in determining relative levels of risk and assessing how the latest information should alter our perception of these levels, if at all.

As two professionals who have been confronted with this problem often, we would encourage the media, in concert with established scientific groups, to establish a reference bureau to "grade" the latest health reports. The public should know, in clear, simple terms, about such things as the quality of research design and the presence or absence of supporting or conflicting research reports. In addition, current reports could be cross-referenced to a "compared-to-what" standard, so the public might have access to meaningful comparisons. One might think of this idea as a United Laboratories test for research and reporting.

For example, news releases periodically frighten us that pesticides in one food or another carry a risk of cancer or genetic mutation. Whenever the news singles out one product for special attention, we should receive comparative information about alleged carcinogenic or mutagenic risk associated with other comparable foods. If a news release were to tell us, for instance, that pesticide residues on apples might cause cancer, we need to know whether apples are the only fruit that have been so identified, whether apples tend to have more pesticide residues than other fruits, or whether all fruits get tainted with pesticide residues in roughly comparable amounts.

A model for this service might be the Food and Drug Administration's ranking of new pharmaceuticals. This is done with criteria designed to help interested parties determine the significance and value of new drugs in the already overflowing medicine cabinet. The FDA continues to tinker with the classification system, but the pre-1992 ranking provides a prototype. Possible ratings include "important therapeutic gain over existing therapies," "modest therapeutic gain," and "little or no therapeutic gain." We see nothing to prevent an independent body from doing the same for scientific releases, helping the interested reader to assess new "health scares": Does this latest press release constitute important new information? Or is it merely an addition to a long string of reports without any apparent lasting value?

The problem of health scares will only get worse as the ability of science to measure and detect continues to evolve. We must develop a mechanism for sorting out true concerns from manufactured ones. The public interest clearly demands it.

Assessing and Accepting Risk

The phenomenal changes in recent decades in science and technology complicate the manner in which we perceive and evaluate risk. The remarkable speedup in data collection, the precision of the data, the evolution of entirely new technologies, the transforming power of the computer—all have changed the way we look at the everyday risks in our lives.

One small but revealing example concerns our ability to detect and measure ever more minute concentrations of just about anything. In the 1950s, for instance, scientists were commonly pleased to measure substances in the human body in concentrations of parts per hundred or parts per thousand. Today, we commonly measure concentrations in parts per million and parts per billion. Will we soon be able to tell how many individual molecules of a substance are inside us? More important, if we do make our detection so accurate, what will we do with the information? We are already inundated by crushing waves of data, and the avalanche has just begun. Our ability to gather information will likely continue to outstrip our ability to make sense of what we accumulate for some time. Not seeing the forest for the trees is no longer the problem. We are in danger of not seeing the forest because of our absorption in the structure of the cells within the trees.

So, as our growing ability to detect low-level risk will reveal some hazard in virtually every conceivable food, beverage, and activity, it is imperative that we apply some meaningful perspective to what we learn and balance that risk with the accompanying benefit.

This is no simple task. Though risk-benefit assessment can appear neutral, most of the fundamental judgments involved depend on the subjective values of the person—bureaucrat or scientist—performing the analysis, with political considerations and pressures hanging like storm clouds over the process. For example, who decides which risks must be balanced against which benefits? Assuming one can easily determine the health risks and benefits, on the one hand, how does one evaluate the weight of such intangibles as pleasure, family, and ethnic traditions? And how does one weigh both of these with freedom of choice, on the other hand? What happens when one segment of the population gets the benefits, whereas another is more likely to experience the risks?

Another difficulty lies in the nature of science: Although simple experiments in a laboratory are often cut-and-dried, real-life data are not. When the research is new, in particular, one can usually find studies to argue both sides of a given issue. Thus the estimates involved in assessing risk depend upon the data selected and which scientists one chooses to produce the data. In controversial matters—and anything related to wine and other alcoholic beverages will inevitably be controversial—competing sides base their contentions on studies carefully selected to illustrate their point.

Clearly, the government's role in risk-benefit assessment is encumbered with potential problems. Yet given the growing role of regulatory agencies in the past decades, the government is sure to dominate the risk-benefit game for the foreseeable future.

We feel it is critical for the government to give the average citizen the freedom of choice by adhering to two principles:

First, the governmental process must favor access to information and education, rather than limiting choices. When government makes complex choices for all, the result will inevitably be unsuitable for many. Most risk assessment situations do not involve either-or choices, in which one choice appears highly risky while another appears to be clearly low-risk. Instead, most choices are characterized by the question, How safe? They are choices in which one seeks greater pleasure or other benefits in return for less safety, or vice versa. Such "how safe?" choices remain inherently difficult, because they depend so heavily on the values of the person making the decision. The government needs to remove itself from "how safe?" choices.

Second, there needs to be a moratorium enforced between each new health scare based upon newly released scientific data and the time when government begins regulatory decision making based on that data. The intelligent lay public understands the incredibly short shelf-life of media-revealed "scientific fact." What we call a dire danger today may mean nothing next year. Though government must be responsive to the needs of the people, the precise nature of those needs cannot be determined on the basis of recent press releases. We need a reasonable lag time in health-related regulation. Everyone involved must recognize that "facts" at our disposal change too quickly.

Warning Labels

Product warning labels serve to inform and educate the consumer. At a practical level, they also offer at least some protection to the manufacturer or producer from liability that might result from failure to warn or failure to inform. But at a subliminal level, warning labels may frighten away consumers who become concerned that a product's risk may outweigh its potential value.

Wine currently carries two types of warning labels. The first, technically an ingredient label, reads, "Contains sulfites." When first mandated in 1986 (see chapter 7), sulfite labels clearly were intended as warning labels to protect potentially allergic patients. Unfortunately, not all sulfite-containing products bear similar labels; other foods and food components with much more serious track records of producing fatal allergic reactions are not required to carry any warnings at all. This inconsistency is an example of an unfortunate and punitive dual standard. While placing exaggerated demands and restrictions on wine suits certain special interest groups, the process ignores the public's more general need for labels that allow informed choice.

TO YOUR HEALTH!

The second label reads: "GOVERNMENT WARNING: (1) According to the Surgeon General, women should not drink alcoholic beverages during pregnancy because of the risk of birth defects. (2) Consumption of alcoholic beverages impairs your ability to drive a car or operate machinery, and may cause health problems."

In applauding the new labels, an official of the National Parent-Teacher Association said, "If a warning label . . . can prevent one death or inform one consumer about the dangers of alcohol consumption, then the law is successful." Such statements certainly carry substantial emotional appeal, but they are a poor basis for effective and sensible public policy. If we want to prevent 1,300 deaths a year, most of them children, why not outlaw bicycles? Or cover them with stickers saying: "GOVERNMENT WARNING FOR PARENTS: Buying this bicycle may lead to serious injury for your child and perhaps even death."

The biggest problem with warning labels is simply that they do not work. The bulk of evidence suggests that "on-product warnings have no measurable impact on user behavior and product safety." In the case of alcoholic beverages, the customary criticisms are (1) heavy drinkers, the ones who are at greatest risk for drunken driving or fetal damage, are least likely to read or pay attention to warning labels; (2) drunken driving and heavy drinking during pregnancy does not correlate with lack of knowledge about dangers related to excessive alcohol consumption; (3) the public already has an extraordinarily high level of awareness (sometimes, in fact, an exaggerated awareness) of health problems related to alcohol; and (4) the labels make absolutely no distinction between use and abuse.

This fourth point is especially relevant to our argument. Though it is true that alcohol "may cause health problems" at high levels of consumption, we have also found that it has distinct benefits at light, regular levels of consumption, and the labels nowhere recognize this fact. If a label is to be used to point out relatively uncommon health risks, why not one to point out much more common health benefits as well?

The most grievous problems with warning labels, from our point of view, is their uselessness in weighing relative risk against relative benefit; as a result, they serve no practical role in decision making. Instead of being a health education tool, warning labels too often become political statements: simplistic, alarming, vague, intended to arouse fear and/or limit product liability.

Though it may seem to some that our fears are exaggerated, consider that a recent California law now requires businesses that sell alcoholic beverages to display a warning that "alcoholic beverages may increase cancer risk." As we saw in chapter 4, alcoholic beverages, *when consumed in excess*, can sometimes increase cancer risk—*in the range of 2 to 3 percent*, according to the Surgeon General. The same Surgeon General's report estimates the increased risk of cancer due to animal fat is in the range of 35 percent (!) yet there is no law in any state that requires meat products and other foods associated with or derived from animal fats to carry a similar label.

TO YOUR HEALTH!

It seems clear that the public would best be served if we first established criteria, applicable to all foods and beverages, about what constitutes appropriate indications for warning labels. Those criteria should then be applied fairly and evenly to all products, without regard to either the political correctness of those products or the political clout of their lobbies.

Of course, removing political considerations from the labeling process may be more easily written about than accomplished, and it may be quite difficult to provide enough information on food labels to make them truly balanced and educational. Still, if product warning labels are to have any value at all, they must differentiate between risks associated with use from those associated with misuse; they must be based on thoroughly documented and uncontroversial data; they must rank risk in some hierarchical form against some familiar standard; and they must be visibly fair in acknowledging health benefits. Without such standards, labels can only be viewed with enormous skepticism and ultimately will serve the public poorly.

TEACH YOUR CHILDREN WELL

If it is important for us as a nation to set responsible public policies, it is critical that we begin this process at home. We must teach our children about the truths concerning the use and abuse of alcohol and especially set for them an example of responsible drinking.

By passing on to its children certain enduring values important to society in the first place, every generation ensures the survival of its fabric. Teaching our youth the intricacies of the "three R's" is essential, but it will not substitute for a strong, thoroughly shared morality. Yet we live in a time in the United States when parents refuse to leave their teenager at home unattended for even one night, fearing the result will be an enormous teenage beer bust hosted by their youngster. Twelve-Step programs occupy meeting rooms all across the country, and one of the fastest growing such programs is Alateen, a Twelve-Step recovery program for teenagers addicted to alcohol.

How is it possible that we have teenagers addicted to alcohol? Despite the fact that it is illegal to sell alcoholic beverages to individuals under the age of twenty-one, most children find they can get alcohol if they are determined. Various surveys show frequent use of alcoholic beverages by high school students, with as many as 40 percent of seniors in high school reporting binge drinking as often as every two weeks; a 1991 survey reported that more than half of fourth through sixth grade students (ages nine to eleven) have used alcohol at least once, and as many as 5 percent identified themselves as "regular drinkers." Not surprisingly, surveys also reveal that children who report a large number of drinking friends, who do not like school, and who attach little significance to the idea of "wrong behavior" are more likely to have drunk to the point of inebriation. And though children who reported a permissive parental attitude toward drinking were very likely to have consumed alcohol at least once, they were less likely to have become drunk than if parental attitudes were restrictive.

This finding gives rise to one of the most important axioms of child development: If you want your children to behave well, be sure you behave well yourself.

The Example of Parents

Especially in the early childhood years, the preschool period, the example of the adults with whom the child lives has such power that other influences fade in importance. If the child grows up in an orderly and peaceful household in which the adults do not abuse each other or the child, he or she is likely to view the world with an optimistic bias as basically a safe place that possesses characteristics of order and structure as a natural condition—even in the face of glimpses of the potential violence in the world, such as dramas acted out on the TV screen every day.

If instead the child lives with adults who fight and abuse each other (or the children) verbally or physically, who drink excessively, who do not take care to be present regularly at bedtime or meals, who do not supervise the child's playtime or television, who leave the child unattended for hours at a time, that child will view the world as a naturally hostile and chaotic place, a place of danger where the unexpected is usually injurious.

Even with the best of upbringings, however, most children experience during their preschool years some sort of failure by their parents that violates their own developing sense of what is right and what is wrong. By the time children enroll in kindergarten, they begin to struggle with the fact that their parents are not always right. Recognizing parental fallibility allows for the substitution of other authorities as sources for distinguishing between right and wrong.

Eventually, at some later point in development, sometime between seven and thirteen, the parents lose their status as the most important and authoritative source for learning. This is usually because as the child grows and matures he or she will examine the important adults in his or her life and will discover any falsehood there; in the face of contradictory information, the child will decide on the basis of which is the more reliable source. From that point forward, the most authoritative source for most children is the peer group. Having discovered parental fallibility, the child gropes for a new standard of authority, and the need to belong may be strong enough to allow the peer group's opinion to substitute for and subvert parental authority.

So, to be effective in shaping the child's worldview and subsequent behavior, the adult caretaker (parent, baby-sitter, or day care supervisor) must be seen as credible by the child. Children must not discover major or basic inconsistencies in what they are told if anything they are told is to be held as truth. Parents who most consistently tell their children the truth will have children who are largely spared the agonizing rebellion and rejection of parental values that seems so much a part of adolescence.

TO YOUR HEALTH!

Another important development that occurs in the pre-school years of almost every American child is the exposure to television. For many the exposure is extensive; but even when limited, television can exert a very powerful influence upon our children's development, some good, some not so good, some quite bad. Though we may never know the full extent of TV's impact upon the young, impressionable mind, we can be sure the effect is a strong and lasting one.

If the parents do not exercise care in choosing what their children may watch, or worse, if they use the TV as an electronic baby-sitter, the new and plastic mind may witness an enormous array of very adult subjects with a monumental overlay of violence, sexual exploitation, and chaos. Of all the features of this very powerful medium, TV commercials carry perhaps the most effect. They are tightly honed to come across with spellbinding power. Many rely heavily on sexual images and sexual innuendo to sell their products.

The wine industry, to its great credit, employs a code of conduct in advertising that forbids the use of sports figures or the suggestion that drinking wine has anything to do with manliness or sexual prowess.

Children may see several thousand of these commercials before enrolling in kindergarten; by the time they are teenagers, the number becomes unfathomable. Few people feel that the effect of such commercials on the developing psyche is neutral or even harmless, but just what contribution they make to the child's eventual worldview, just how much more or less a complete person they may make him or her, remains unanswered, at least for now.

Still, it is commonly felt that the overall effect of early childhood television is to trivialize in the minds of preschoolers the major moral and social questions of our civilization. In addition to these types of commercials, violence and death on television are so commonplace, divorce and broken families so natural, lying, stealing, double dealing, cursing, and drug trafficking so much a part of the daily fare, that the distinction between right and wrong can be washed away in electronic images.

Our children desperately need credible adult caretakers who will steer them away from so much of the daily TV and movie fare and who will patiently point out to them that, even in the real life of a private detective in a big city, it is rare to be shot at, or to be beaten up, or to encounter a corpse in a dumpster. In the real life of doctors and nurses at the hospital, having illicit sex in the X-ray suite or operating room lounge is the exception rather than the rule.

The School's Role

As pervasive as it may seem to some of us, television is obviously not the only extrafamilial influence in our children's lives. School plays an enormous role in the life of almost every child in this country. Thus, just as the parents of young children establish their credentials by being truthful, in the early days of school, teachers have an opportunity to establish a reliable, credible institutional authority. Children who do not believe in the reliability or credibility of the schools, which represents their first exposure to institutional authority, may have trouble dealing with the many institutional systems they will face throughout their lives.

To the extent that schoolteachers promulgate half-truths or total falsehoods, children are liable to reject the values of institutional authority when they discover the truth on their own. When schools teach that "Just say no" is the only safe approach in dealing with the availability of drugs, and that drinking wine with dinner constitutes an example of drug abuse, children will likely go along with it at first. But as they get older and discover that the answers to these issues are not as simple as "just say no," when they observe parents and other adults having wine with meals, or when they themselves have an illicit taste of beer and find they are not suddenly transformed into an addict, they will be more likely to reject other "truths" learned in school. They will be more likely to develop the cynical attitude toward the adult world that is all too prevalent among today's youth.

Perhaps the worst consequence of all this is the loss of reliable authority. When kids observe peers apparently safely having a marijuana cigarette or hear a friend describing the wonderful "high" that results from smoking crack cocaine, it should come as no surprise if they decide that a conspiracy of misinformation exists surrounding drug use and that they have to discover the truth for themselves.

TEACH YOUR CHILDREN

The most reliable witnesses become their peer group; they rightly question the validity of the *entire* scheme of values their parents and teachers hold because they have determined certain specific, identifiable elements of that scheme to be false.

Sadly, in spite of a great deal of research to support these conclusions, professional alcohol control groups continue to work hard to eliminate the concept of responsible use. These groups, headed by President Bush's Surgeon General, Dr. Novella, sought to define any use of alcoholic beverages as equivalent to drug abuse. This flies in the face of the majority of current research and completely contradicts the empirical wisdom of history as well as modern cultural opinion.

In this culturally diverse society, millions of families regard daily wine consumption as nothing more than one more element in a meal. Why then adopt an official governmental strategy that calls upon our nation's schoolteachers to brand these families as abusive, to undermine the valuable benefits of cultural heritage proven by history? In an already confusing world, shared family experiences can serve to stabilize and provide reference for the developing child. Why not teach acceptance of and respect for safe parental behaviors rather than vilifying them?

The Importance of Truth

As a general rule, the greater the misinformation touted by authorities, the greater will be the loss of confidence in authority when the truth finally surfaces. For example, educators and most people doing alcohol research in the United States teach that any alcohol use by children is dangerous. They also hold that alcohol use by individuals under age twenty-one carries an even greater risk than for adults. However, the fact is that for thousands of years many Mediterranean and other European peoples commonly gave their children wine with meals (usually diluted with water or seltzer) from the earliest days of childhood—without ill effect. For some, this practice continues today without the least hint that it leads to a high incidence of adult alcoholism. In fact, the predominantly wine-drinking districts of the Mediterranean countries consistently show the least problems associated with abusive alcohol consumption (a relatively high level of alcoholism among the French tends to be confined to the urban areas of northern France, where consumption of high-proof spirits is more common). Similarly, among religious Jews, ritual exposure to alcohol from age thirteen on does not lead to increased troubles with alcohol abuse. In fact, Jews in traditional cultures do not show *any* appreciable risk for alcoholism.

In light of these facts, it seems only logical that, instead of concluding children and alcohol to be a dangerous mix, we should look to see what is different about the way American children consume alcohol. The answer is obvious, and it is hard to believe there is not more recognition of it in this country: Whereas children from the countries mentioned above first discover alcohol in a relatively light form—generally wine and usually diluted—with the approbation and guidance of adults, drinking in a responsible, family setting, most American children come by alcohol as an illicit substance, sneaked out away from parents or any other figure of responsible authority.

Recently one of us met the son of a teetotaling family from the Midwest who was taught as a child that alcohol must be entirely avoided on moral and religious grounds. He told us that when the children in his family were old enough to escape parental control, all but one quickly "went wild," engaging in excessive alcohol consumption, resulting in alcoholism and patterns of abuse. This was not the first time we had heard such a story.

So, when our children eventually get around to trying a drink, as research consistently confirms the vast majority of them will do despite the steady drumbeat of the "just say no" message, and they find it does them no noticeable immediate harm, several things can happen. First, the basic credibility of the teaching authorities may be tarnished because experience contradicts the simplistic official message. Second, children may find themselves in a conspiratorial isolation from adults in authority. This alienation makes less likely a productive general discussion with parents and other adults. Third, in violating authority, they have done something thrilling and dangerous; they are much more likely to attach significance to the experience and therefore much more likely to drink excessively at some point in the future. Finally, some will experience a harmful feeling of guilt and a loss of self-esteem because of violating one of the high-profile rules of our society. Various research studies have shown that these feelings predispose one to a future pattern of abuse. In fact, one article reported that all sorts of damaging social behaviors among teenagers increased as alcohol became increasingly less available—a feature the authors referred to as "the forbidden fruit syndrome."

What We Must Do

If we love our children, we owe them our best efforts to protect them from the very real dangers of this world. Most important, we need to teach them, so far as we are able, values and concepts that will help them in choosing a safe and morally defensible direction at every crossroad.

As loving parents, we must do our best to be role models for responsible living; if our lives include the healthy use of wine with meals, we should be able to discuss this with them and perhaps to include them, even in childhood, by serving small or diluted samples of wine with dinner as other cultures have done for centuries. We should discuss with our children the complexity of the contradictory messages they get at school and in other venues about alcohol consumption.

If our lives do not include the use of alcohol, we must nevertheless be able to discuss rationally and calmly the elements of risk and the potential benefits involved in drinking wine or other alcoholic beverages. At all costs we must guard against teaching our children as facts things we do not know to be true. Whether we use alcohol or not, we must recognize that our children will soon be adults in a world in which the vast majority of people drink alcohol in some form; we owe them some preparation for that fact. And we must recognize that our children will ultimately decide for themselves whether they will drink, despite what we believe or attempt to teach.

If we teach our children to avoid simplistic slogans as substitutes for reasoned analysis, to approach complex problems with an open mind free of rigid dogma; if we teach them the great value of shared family experience and model for them a life lived in moderation; if they learn the importance of mutual respect and acceptance of others in our culturally diverse nation, they will be less likely to fall prey to drug or alcohol addiction; they will be less likely to live in chaos, and less likely to be involved in abusive relationships.

If we do not seek every opportunity to tell them the truth so far as we know it, they will find some other source they can believe (most often their teenage peer group). If we do not take care to provide them with a solid example of a life well lived, as free as possible from deceit or falsehood, we run the risk of guaranteeing their rejection of all our teachings, all our values, isolating them from our counsel and exposing them to the dangers of facing a world for which they are unprepared

Our children's health and success in life depend dramatically upon whether we teach them or preach to them, whether we tell the truth or spout dogma, whether we trust them enough to give them freedom or keep them rigidly under control, whether we enfold them or alienate them, whether we help them learn from their mistakes or blame them for these; most important, our children's ultimate success depends strongly upon the model for moderate behavior and truthfulness they see in us.

TEACH YOUR CHILDREN

Final Note

Not everyone approves of wine or other alcoholic beverages, and if past history is any judge, there never will be a time when wine wins the approval of everyone. But the vast majority of people worldwide consume alcohol in some form or another, and that statistic is likely to be valid for as long as there are people to eat and drink. Most consumers drink responsibly and healthfully, without deleterious consequences, especially when they drink wine.

We need public policy that recognizes these facts and treats them respectfully. To limit unwelcome behavior from the abusive minority, we need rules and regulations directed at the specific undesired behaviors, not rules directed at the beverage that the majority use to healthful advantage.

Bibliography & Resources

INTRODUCTION

Gordis, E. "Alcohol Use and Abuse: Where Do the Numbers Come From?" *Alcohol Alert*. National Institute on Alcohol Abuse and Alcoholism (NIAAA). January 1990.
Longnecker, M.P., and B. MacMahon. "Associations between Alcoholic Beverage Consumption and Hospitalization, 1983 National Health Interview Survey." *Am J Pub Health* 78(1988):153–56.

CHAPTER 1: WINE AND NUTRITION

Gershoff, S. *The Tufts University Guide to Total Nutrition*. New York: Harper & Row, 1990.
Gruchow, Harvey W., et al. "Alcohol Consumption, Nutrient Intake and Relative Body Weight among US Adults." *Am J Clin Nutr* 42(1985): 289–95.

Kant, A. K., et al. "Dietary Diversity in the US Population, NHANES II, 1976–1980." *J Am Diet Assoc* 91(1991):1526–31.

National Research Council. *Recommended Dietary Allowances.* 10th ed. Washington, D.C.: National Academy Press, 1989.

Pennington, J. A. T. *Food Values of Portions Commonly Used.* 15th ed. New York: Harper & Row, 1989.

Scott, F. W. "Cow's Milk and Insulin-dependent Diabetes Mellitus: Is There a Relationship?" *Am J Clin Nutr* 51(1990):489–91.

U.S. Dept. of Health and Human Services (USDHHS). *The Surgeon General's Report on Nutrition and Health.* Washington, D.C.: GPO, 1988.

CHAPTER 2: WINE AND THE HEART

Anderson, P., et al. "What Are Safe Levels of Alcohol Consumption?" *Br Med J* 289(1984):1657–58.

Blackwelder, et al. "Alcohol and Mortality: The Honolulu Heart Study." *Am J Med* 68(1980):164–69.

Boffetta, P., and L. Garfinkel. "Alcohol Drinking and Mortality among Men Enrolled in an American Cancer Society Prospective Study." *Epidemiol* 1[5](Sept. 1990):342–48.

Camargo, C., et al. "The Effect of Moderate Alcohol Intake on Serum Apolipoproteins A-I and A-II." *JAMA* 253[19](1985):2854–57.

Ciampricotti, R., et al. "Myocardial Infarction and Sudden Death after Sport: Acute Coronary Angiographic Findings." *Cathet Cardiovasc Diagn* 17(1989):193–97.

Driscoll, C. E., and G. Nelson. "Not Just a Man's Disease." *The Female Patient* 17(June 1992):11–14.

Ellison, R. C. "Cheers!" *Epidemiol* (Sept. 1990):1[5]:337–39.

Frankel, E. N., et al. "Inhibition of Oxidation of Human Low-Density Lipoprotein by Phenolic Substances in Red Wine." *Lancet* (Feb. 1993):341.

Garg, R., et al. "Alcohol Consumption and Risk of Ischemic Heart Disease in Women." *Arch Intern Med* 153(1993):1211–16.

Gordon, T. K., "Drinking and Mortality: The Framingham Study." *Am J Epidemiol* 120[1](June 1984):97–107.

Gordon, T., et al. "High Density Lipoprotein as a Protective Factor Against Coronary Heart Disease. The Framingham Study." *Am J Med* 62(1977):707–14.

Holden, C., ed. "Low-lipid Blues." *Science* 259(Jan. 1993):460.

Kaplan, N. M. "Bashing Booze: The Danger of Losing the Benefits of Moderate Alcohol Consumption." Part 1. *Am Heart J* 121[6](June 1991):1854–56.

Kinsella, J., et al. "Inhibition In Vitro of Oxidation of Human Low-density Lipoproteins by Phenolic Substances in Wine." *Lancet* (Feb. 1993): 342.

Klag, M. J., et al. "Serum Cholesterol in Young Men and Subsequent Cardiovascular Disease." *NEJM* 328[5](Feb. 1993):313–18.

Klatsky, A. "Correlates of Alcohol Beverage Preference: Traits of Persons Who Choose Wine, Liquor, or Beer." *Br Med J* (1990):85.

Klatsky, A., and M. Armstrong. "Alcoholic Beverage Choice and Risk of Coronary Artery Disease Mortality: Do Red Wine Drinkers Fare Best?" *Am J Cardiol* (Feb. 1993):71.

Klatsky, A., et al. "Alcohol and Mortality: A Ten Year Kaiser-Permanente Experience." *Ann Intern Med* 95[2](1981):139–45.

———. "Alcohol and Mortality." *Ann Intern Med* 117[8](1992):646–54.

———. "Relations of Alcoholic Beverage Use to Subsequent Coronary Artery Disease Hospitalization." *Am J Cardiol* 58[9](1986):710–14.

Kono, S., et al. "The Relationship Between Alcohol and Mortality Among Japanese Physicians." *Int J Epidemiol* 4(Dec. 1983):437–41.

Kreutz, J. M., and J. E. Mazuzan. "Sudden Asystole in a Marathon Runner: The Athletic Heart Syndrome and Its Anesthetic Implications." *Anesthesiology* 73[6](Dec. 1990):1266–68.

LaPorte, R., et al. "The Relation of Alcohol to Coronary Heart Disease and Mortality: Implications for Public Health Policy." *J Pub Hlth Plcy* 1[3](1980):198–223.

———. "Alcohol, Coronary Heart Disease, and Total Mortality." *Recent Dev Alcohol* 3(1985):157–63.

Lieber, C. "To Drink (Moderately) or Not to Drink?" *NEJM* 310[13] (1984):846–48.

Manninen, V., et al. "Lipid Alterations and Decline in the Incidence of Coronary Heart Disease in the Helsinki Heart Study." *JAMA* 260(1988):641–51.

Manson, J., et al. "The Primary Prevention of Myocardial Infarction." *NEJM* 326[21](May 1992):1406–16.

Morgan, R. E., et al. "Plasma Cholesterol and Depressive Symptoms in Older Men." *Lancet* 341(Jan. 1993):75–79.

Myerburg, R. J., et al. "Sudden Cardiac Death: Structure, Function, and Time-dependence of Risk." Suppl. 1. *Circulation* 81[1](Jan. 1992): I-2-I-10.

Nanji, A. "Alcohol and Ischemic Heart Disease: Wine, Beer, or Both?" *Int J Cardiol* 8(1985):487–89.

National Institute on Alcohol Abuse and Alcoholism. "Moderate Drinking." *Alcohol Alert* 16(Apr. 1992):315.

Renaud, S., and M. De Lorgeril. "Wine, Alcohol, Platelets and the French Paradox for Coronary Heart Disease." *Lancet* (June 1992):339.

Rimm, M. J., et al. "Vitamin E Consumption and the Risk of Coronary Heart Disease in Men." *NEJM* 328(May 1993):1450–56.

Seigneur, M., et al. "Effect of the Consumption of Alcohol, White Wine, and Red Wine on Platelet Function and Serum Lipids." *J Appl Cardiol* (1990):5.

Shaper, A. G. "Alcohol and Mortality: A Review of Prospective Studies." *Br J Addic* (1990):85.

———. "Alcohol, the Heart, and Health." *Am J Pub Hlth* 83(1993):6.

Siemann, E., and L. Creasy. "Concentration of the Phytoalexin Resveratrol in Wine." *Am J Enol Viticult* 43(1992):1.

Siscovick, D. S., et al. "Moderate Alcohol Consumption and Primary Cardiac Arrest." *Am J Epidemiol* 123(1986):499–503.

St. Leger, A., et al. "Factors Associated with Cardiac Mortality in Developed Countries with Particular Reference to the Consumption of Wine." *Lancet* 1(May 1979):1016–17.

Stampfer, M., et al. "Prospective Study of Moderate Alcohol Consumption and the Risk of Coronary Disease and Stroke in Women." *NEJM* 319(1988):5.

———. "Vitamin E Consumption and the Risk of Coronary Disease in Women." *NEJM* 328(May 1993):1444–49.

Testa, M., et al. "Quality of Life and Antihypertensive Therapy in Men." *NEJM* 328[13](Apr. 1993):907–21.

USDHHS. "Implications for Public Health Policy: Coronary Heart Disease." *Surgeon General's Report on Health and Nutrition*. Rockville, MD: USDHHS, 1989.

Valle, G. A., et al. "An Acute Cardiovascular Event in an Endurance-trained Athlete." *Heart Lung* 17[2](Mar. 1988):216–22.

Wenger, N., et al. "Cardiovascular Health and Disease in Women." *NEJM* 329[4](1993):247–56.

Yano, et al. "Ten Year Incidence of Coronary Heart Disease in the Honolulu Heart Program." *Am J Epidemiol* 119[5](1984):653–66.

CHAPTER 3: WINE AND THE DIGESTIVE TRACT

Achord, J. L. "Nutrition, Alcohol, and the Liver." *Am J Gastroent* 83[3] (Mar. 1988):244–48.

Carbone, J., et al. "The Effect of Wine in Decompensated Hepatic Cirrhosis." *J Clin Invest* 36(1957):878.

D'Houtard, A., et al. "Alcohol Consumption in France: Production, Consumption, Morbidity, and Mortality—Prevention and Education in the Last Three Decades." *Ad Alc Sub Abuse* 8(1989):1.

Dickerson, W., and D. A. Muscatine, eds. *Medical and Therapeutic Values*. Chap. 8. Berkeley: Univ. of California Press, 1984.

DuPont, H.L. "How Safe Is the Food We Eat?" *JAMA* 268(Dec. 1992):3240.

Friedman, G. D., et al. "Cigarettes, Alcohol, Coffee, and Peptic Ulcer." *NEJM* 290(1974):469.

Green, G. A. "Gastrointestinal Disorders in the Athlete." *Clin Sports Med* 11[2](Apr. 1992):453–70.

Groover, J. R. "Alcoholic Liver Disease." *Emer Med Clin North Am* 8[4](Nov. 1990):887–902.

Jost, J., et al. "Comparison of Dietary Patterns between Population Samples in the Three French MONICA Nutritional Surveys." *Rev Epidemiol et Sante Publ* 38(1990):517–23.

Lereboullet, J. "Variations of Alcohol Level in the Blood Depending on the Beverage Drunk." *Bull Acad Nat Med* 154(1970):433–47.

Lieber, C. S. "Biochemical and Molecular Basis of Alcohol-induced Injury to Liver and Other Tissues." *NEJM* 319[25](Dec. 1988):1639–50.

Lolli, G., and M. Rubin. "The Effect of Concentration of Alcohol on the Rate of Absorption and the Shape of the Blood Alcohol Curve." *Quart J Stud Alc* 4(1963):57–63.

MacMath, T. L. "Alcohol and Gastrointestinal Bleeding." *Emer Med Clin North Am* 8[4](Nov. 1990):859–72.

Murdock, H. R. "Blood Glucose and Alcohol Levels after Administration of Wine to Human Subjects." *Am J Clin Nutr* 24(1971):394–96.

O'Connor, M. "Europe and Nutrition: Prospects for Public Health." *Br Med J* 304(Jan. 1992):178–80.

Scholten, P. "Spirits, Wine, and Beer Consumption in Relation to Cirrhosis Mortality in the US." *Bull Med Friends of Wine* 30(Feb. 1988):1.

Schumsinger, W. H. "Alcohol Protects Against Cholesterol Gallstone Formation." *Surgery* 207(1988):641–47.

Smart, R., et al. "Factors in Recent Reductions in Liver Cirrhosis Deaths." *J Stud Alc* 52(1991):3.

Summerskill, W. H., et al. "Response to Alcohol in Chronic Alcoholics with Liver Disease." *Lancet* 272(1957):335–40.

USDHHS. "Gastrointestinal Diseases." *Surgeon General's Report on Health and Nutrition.* Rockville, MD: USDHHS.

Valencia-Parparcen, J. "Alcoholic Gastritis." *Clin Gastro* 10[2](1981): 389–99.

Walker, A. "Drinking Water—Doubts about Quality." *Br Med J* 304(Jan. 1992):175–78.

CHAPTER 4: CANCER

Aaltonen, L. A., et al. "Clues to the Pathogenesis of Familial Colorectal Cancer. *Science* 260(May 1993):812–16.

Bouchardy, C., et al. "Alcohol, Beer, and Cancer of the Pancreas." *Int J Cancer* 45(1990):5.

Castillo, M. H., et al. "The Effects of the Bioflavonoid Quercetin on Squamous Cell Carcinoma of Head and Neck Origin." *Am J Surg* 158[4](Oct. 1989):351–55.

Doll, R., and R. Peto. "The Causes of Cancer: Quantitative Estimates of Avoidable Risks of Cancer in the United States Today." *J Nat Cancer Inst* 66(1981):1191.

Gapstur, S. M., et al. "Increased Risk of Breast Cancer with Alcohol Consumption in Postmenopausal Women." *Am J Epidemiol* 136[10](Nov. 1992):1222–31.

Gorman, C., and U. Plon. "Danger Overhead." *Time*, October 1992, 70.

Harris, J. R., et al. "Breast Cancer." Part 3. *NEJM* 327[7](Aug. 1992): 473–80.

Howe, G., et al. "The Association between Alcohol and Breast Cancer Risk: Evidence from the Combined Analysis of Six Dietary Control Studies." *Int J Cancer* 47[5](1991):707–10.

Jun-mo Nam, J. K., et al. "Cigarette Smoking, Alcohol, and Nasopharyngeal Carcinoma: A Case-control Study among U.S. Whites." *J Nat Cancer Inst* 84[8](Apr. 1992):619–22.

Kohlmeier, L., et al. "Pet Birds as an Independent Risk Factor for Lung Cancer: Case-control Study." *Br Med J* 305(Oct. 1992):986–89.

Kune, G. A., and L. Vitetta. "Alcohol Consumption and the Etiology of Colorectal Cancer: a Review of the Scientific Evidence from 1957 to 1991." *Nutr Cancer* 18[2](1992):97–111.

Leighton, T. "Quercetin as a Cancer Preventative." *Bull Soc Med Friends of Wine* 32(June 1990):1.

Li, F.P. "Cancer Epidemiology and Prevention." In *Medicine*. New York: Scientific American, 1988.

Longnecker, M. P., et al. "A Meta-analysis of Alcohol Consumption in Relation to Breast Cancer." *JAMA* 260(1988):652–56.

Marx, J. "Learning How to Suppress Cancer." *Science* 261(Sept. 1993): 1385–87.

Peltomaki, P., et al. "Genetic Mapping of a Locus Predisposing to Human Colorectal Cancer." *Science* 260(May 1993):810–12.

Ranelletti, F. O., et al. "Growth-inhibitory Effect of Quercetin and Presence of Type-II Estrogen-binding Sites in Human Colon-cancer Cell Lines and Primary Colorectal Tumors." *Int J Cancer* 50[3](Feb. 1992):486–92.

Seitz, H. K., et al. "Gastrointestinal Carcinogenesis: Ethanol as a Risk Factor." *Eur J Cancer Prev* 1 Suppl. 3(Oct. 1992):5–18.

Slattery, M. L., et al. "Tobacco, Alcohol, Coffee, and Caffeine as Risk Factors for Colon Cancer in a Low Risk Population." *Epidemiol* 1[2](1990):141–45.

Stone, R. "Polarized Debate: EMF's and Cancer." *Science* 258(Nov. 1992):1724–25.

BIBLIOGRAPHY & RESOURCES

USDHHS. *Diet, Nutrition and Cancer Prevention: The Good News.* Bethesda, MD: National Cancer Institute, 1987.

———. *Surgeon General's Report on Health and Nutrition.* Rockville, MD: USDHHS, 1988.

———. *What You Need to Know about Cancer.* Bethesda, MD: National Cancer Institute, 1989.

Varmus, H. "Oncogenes and Transcriptional Control." *Science* 238(Dec. 1987):1337–39.

Weinberg, R. A. "Oncogenes and the Mechanisms of Carcinogenesis."In *Medicine.* New York: Scientific American, 1990.

CHAPTER 5: WOMEN AND WINE

Abel, E. L., et al. "A Revised Conservative Estimate of the Incidence of FAS and Its Economic Impact." *Alc Clin Exp Res* 15[3](June 1991): 514–24.

Alpert, J. J., and B. Zuckerman. "Alcohol Use during Pregnancy: What Is the Risk?" *Ped Rev* 12[12](June 1991):375–81.

Alpert, J. J., et al. "Maternal Alcohol Consumption and Newborn Assessment: Methodology of the Boston City Hospital Prospective Study." *Neurobehav Toxicol Teratol* 3[2](June 1981):195–201.

Ames, B. N., et al. "Nature's Chemicals and Synthetic Chemicals: Comparative Toxicology." *Proc Nat Acad Sci USA* 87(Oct. 1990): 7782–86.

Annas, G. P. "Protecting the Liberty of Pregnant Patients." *NEJM* 316[19](May 1987):1213–14.

Artal, R. "Exercise and Pregnancy." *Clin Sports Med* 11[2](Apr. 1992):363–77.

Astley, S. J., et al. "Analysis of Facial Shape in Children Gestationally Exposed to Marijuana, Alcohol, and/or Cocaine." *Pediatrics* 89[1](Jan. 1992:67–77.

Autti-Ramo, I., et al. "The Effect of Intrauterine Alcohol Exposure in Various Durations on Early Cognitive Development." *Neuropediatrics* 22[4](1991):203–10.

Bell, N. K. "Maternal Substance Abuse: A Daunting Task for Society." *Med Ethics* 7[3](July 1992):6–7.

Blume, S. B. "Women and Alcohol: A Review." *JAMA* 256[11](Sept. 1986):1467–70.

Cnattingius, S., et al. "Delayed Childbearing and Risk of Adverse Perinatal Outcome: A Population Based Study." *JAMA* 268[7](Aug. 1992): 886—90.

Colditz, G. A., et al. "Family History, Age, and Risk of Breast Cancer: Prospective Data from the Nurses' Health Study." *JAMA* 270[3](July 1993):338–43.

Cook, P. S., R. C. Peterson, and D. T. Moore. *Alcohol, Tobacco, and Other Drugs May Harm the Unborn.* Rockville, MD: USDHHS, 1990.

Folsom, A. R., et al. "Body Fat Distribution and 5-year Risk of Death in Older Women." *JAMA* 269(Jan. 1993):483–87.

Forrest, F., et al. "Reported Social Alcohol Consumption during Pregnancy and Infants' Development at 18 Months." *Br Med J* 303[6793](1991):22–26.

Gannett News Service. "Genes May Predispose Women to Alcoholism." *Marin Independent Journal,* October 1992, sec. A1.

Gavaler, J. S. "The Association between Moderate Alcoholic Beverage Consumption and Serum Levels of Estradiol in Normal Postmenopausal Women." *J Stud Alc* 53(1992):4.

Gavaler, J. S., et al. "The Association between Moderate Alcoholic Beverage Consumption and Serum Estradiol and Testosterone Levels in Normal Postmenopausal Women: Relationship to the Literature." *Alc Clin Exp Res* 16[1](Feb. 1992):87–92.

Giovanucci, E., et al. "Folate, Methionine, and Alcohol Intake and Risk of Colorectal Adenoma." *J Nat Cancer Inst* 86(1993):11.

Harvey, E. B., et al. "Alcohol Consumption and Breast Cancer." *J Nat Cancer Inst* 78(1987):657–61.

Hiatt, H., et al. "Alcohol Consumption and the Risk of Breast Cancer in a Prepaid Health Plan." *Cancer Res* 48(Apr. 1988):2284–87.

Hoyme, H. E. "Teratogenically Induced Fetal Anomalies." *Clin Perinat* 17[3](Sept. 1990):547–67.

International Agency for Research on Cancer (IARC). "Monograph on Alcohol and Cancer." October 1987.

Jason, J. "Breast-feeding in 1991." *NEJM* 324[14](Oct. 1991):1036–38.

Jones, K. L., et al. "Pattern of Malformation in Offspring of Chronic Alcoholic Mothers." *Lancet* 1(1973):1267.

Kaminsky, M., et al. "Alcohol Use and Pregnancy and Fetal Growth." *J Epidemiol Comm Health* 9(1990):3.

Kessler, L. G. "The Relationship between Age and Incidence of Breast Cancer." *Cancer* 69(1992):1896–903.

Knupfer, G. "Abstaining for Fetal Health: The Fiction That Even Light Drinking Is Dangerous." *Br J Addic* 9(1991):1063–73.

La Vecchia, C., et al. "Alcohol Consumption and the Risk of Breast Cancer in Women." *J Nat Cancer Inst* 75(1983):61–65.

Lee, J. "Screening and Informed Consent." *NEJM* 328[6](Feb. 1993): 438–40.

Little, R., et al. "Maternal Alcohol Use during Breastfeeding and Infant Mental and Motor Development at One Year." *NEJM* 321(1989): 425–30.

Little, R. E., and J. K. Wendt. "The Effects of Maternal Drinking in the Reproductive Period: An Epidemiologic Review." *J Subst Abuse* 3[2](1991):187–204.

Los Angeles Times Wire Service. "Mothers-to-be Warned to Avoid Hot Tubs, Spas." *San Jose Mercury News*, August 1992, sec. 1A.

Marshall, E. "Search for a Killer: Focus Shifts from Fat to Hormones." *Science* (January 1993):259.

Martin-Moreno, J. M., et al. "Alcoholic Beverage Consumption and Risk of Breast Cancer in Spain." *Cancer Causes and Controls* (June 1993):4.

Massachusetts Medical Society. "Pregnancy Risks Determined from Birth Certificate Data—United States, 1989." *MMWR* 41[30](July 1992):556–63.

May, P. A. "Fetal Alcohol Effects among North American Indians." *Alc Health Res World* 15[3](1991):239–48.

Mettlin, C. "Breast Cancer Risk Factors: Contributions to Planning Breast Cancer Control." *Cancer* 69(1992):1904–10.

Mills, G., et al. "Maternal Alcohol Consumption and Birthweight—How Much Drinking in Pregnancy Is Safe?" *JAMA* 252[14](1984):1875–79.

Milunskey, A., et al. "Maternal Heat Exposure and Neural Tube Defects." *JAMA* 268[7](Aug. 1992):882–85.

Nanji, A. A., et al. "Increased Susceptibility of Women to Alcohol: Is Beer the Reason?" *NEJM* 213[9](Feb. 1985):585.

Painter, K. "Heart Disease: Women's Hidden Killer." *Marin Independent Journal*, February 1993, sec. D8.

Peacock, J. L., et al. "Effects on Birthweight of Alcohol and Caffeine Consumption in Smoking Women." *J Epidemiol Comm Health* 45(1991):159–63.

Reichman, M., et al. "Effects of Alcohol Consumption on Plasma and Urinary Hormone Concentrations in Premenopausal Women." *J Nat Cancer Inst* 85[9](1993).

Roman, P. M. "Biological Features of Women's Alcohol Use: A Review." *Public Health Rep* 103[6](Nov. 1988):628–37.

Rosett, H. L., and L. Weiner. "Alcohol and Pregnancy: A Clinical Perspective." *Ann Rev Med* 36(1985):73–80.

Rosett, H. L., et al. "Patterns of Alcohol Consumption and Fetal Development." *Obstet Gynecol* 61[5](May 1983):539–46.

———. "Reduction of Alcohol Consumption during Pregnancy with Benefits to the Newborn." *Alcohol Clin Exp Res* 4[2](Apr. 1980):178–84.

———. "Treatment Experience with Pregnant Problem Drinkers." *JAMA* 249[15](Apr. 1983):2029–33.

Saunders, J. B., et al. "Do Women Develop Alcoholic Liver Disease More Readily Than Men?" *Br Med J* 282(1981):1140–43.

Schatzkin, A., et al. "Alcohol Consumption and Breast Cancer: A Cross-national Correlation Study.' *Int J Epidemiol* 18[1](1989):28–31.

Streissguth, A. P., et al. "Moderate Prenatal Alcohol Exposure: Effects on Child IQ and Learning Problems at Age 7 1/2 Years." *Alc Clin Exp Res* 14[5](Oct. 1990):662–69.

Talmamini, R., et al. "Social Factors, Diet and Breast Cancer in a Northern Italian Population." *Breast Cancer J* 49(1984):723–29.

———. "Fetal Alcohol Syndrome and Other Effects of Alcohol on Pregnancy Outcome." *Seventh Special Report to the U.S. Congress on Alcohol and Health.* Rockville, MD: USDHHS, 1990.

———. "Maternal and Child Nutrition." *The Surgeon General's Report on Health and Nutrition* Washington, D.C.: GPO, 1988.

Vega, W. A., et al. "Prevalence and Magnitude of Perinatal Substance Exposures in California." *NEJM* 329[12](Sept. 1993):850–54.

Walpole, I., et al. "Low to Moderate Maternal Alcohol Use before and during Pregnancy, and Neurobehavioral Outcome in the Newborn Infant." *Dev Med Child Neurol* 33[10](Oct. 1991):875–83.

Willett, W. C., et al. "Moderate Alcohol Consumption and Risk of Breast Cancer." *NEJM* 316[19](1987):1174–80.

CHAPTER 6: WINE AND MENTAL ABILITY

Alterman, Arthur I., and Julia G. Hall. "Effects of Social Drinking and Familial Alcoholism Risk on Cognitive Functioning: Null Findings." *Alc Clin Exp Res* 13(1989):799–803.

Baum-Baicker, Cynthia. "The Psychological Benefits of Moderate Alcohol Consumption: A Review of the Literature." *Drug and Alcohol Dependence* 15(1985):305–22.

Best, M. L. *Compendium of Drug Therapy.* Secaucus: Compendium Publications Group, 1993.

Kastenbaum, R. "Prevention of Age-related Problems." In *Handbook of Clinical Gerontology,* edited by L. L. Carstensen and B. Edelstein. New York: Pergamon Press, 1988.

MacArthur, Rodger D., and Robert Sekuler. "Alcohol and Motion Perception." *Perception and Psychophysics* 31(1982):502–05.

Moscowitz, H., et al. "Skills Performance at Low Blood Alcohol Levels." *J Stud Alc* 46(1985):482–85.

Parsons, O. A. "Cognitive Functioning in Sober Social Drinkers: A Review and Critique." *J Stud Alc* 47(1986):101–14.

Robertson, Ian. "Does Moderate Drinking Cause Mental Impairment?" *Br Med J* 289(1984):711–12.

Starmer, Graham A. "Effects of Low to Moderate Doses of Ethanol on Human Driving-related Performance." In *Human Metabolism of Alcohol*, vol. 1, edited by Kathryn E. Crow and Richard D. Batt. Boca Raton, FL: CRC Press, 1984.

Wilson, James R., and Robert Plomin. "Individual Differences in Sensitivity and Tolerance to Alcohol." *Social Biology* 32(1985): 162–84.

CHAPTER 7:
CONTAMINANTS AND ADDITIVES IN WINE

Brostoff, J., and S. J. Challacombe. *Food Allergy and Intolerance.* London: Bailliere Tindall, 1987.

Bureau of Alcohol, Tobacco, and Firearms. "Report of Analyses of Wines and Related Products to Determine Lead Content." Washington, D.C.: Dept. of the Treasury, 1991.

Eastaugh, Janet, and Suzanne Shepherd. "Infectious and Toxic Syndromes from Fish and Shellfish Consumption: A Review." *Arch Intern Med* 149(1989):1735–40.

Goldberg, S. J., et al. "An Association of Human Congenital Cardiac Malformations and Drinking Water Contaminants." *J Am Coll Cardiol* 16(1990):155–64.

Gunderson, Ellis L. *FDA Total Diet Study, April 1982-April 1986, Dietary Intakes of Pesticides, Selected Elements, and Other Chemicals.* Washington, D.C.: FDA, 1986.

Jacobus, C. H., et al. "Hypervitaminosis D Associated with Drinking Milk." *NEJM* 326(1992):1173–77.

Litovitz, Toby L., et al. "1989 Annual Report of the American Association of Poison Control Centers National Data Collection System." *Am J Emer Med* 8(1990):394–442.

Mathison, D. A., D. D. Stevenson, and R. A. Simon. "Precipitating Factors in Asthma—Aspirin, Sulfites, and Other Drugs and Chemicals." *Chest* Suppl. 87(1985):50–54.

Russell, H. H., et al. "Chemical Contamination of California Drinking Water." *West J Med* 147(1987):615–22.

Ryan, C. A., et al. "Massive Outbreak of Antimicrobial-resistant Salmonellosis Traced to Pasteurized Milk." *JAMA* 258(1987):3269–74.

Waites, W. M., and J. P. Arbuthnott. "Foodborne Illness: An Overview." *Lancet* 336(1990):722–25.

Yunginger, J. W., et al. "Fatal Food-induced Anaphylaxis." *JAMA* 260 (1988):1450–52.

CHAPTER 8: ALCOHOLISM, ABUSE,
AND THE PERCEPTION OF RISK

Brownell, K. "Dieting and the Search for the Perfect Body: Where Physiology and Culture Collide." *Behav Res Ther* 22(1991):1–12.

Bush, B., et al. "Screening for Alcohol Abuse Using the CAGE Questionnaire." *Am J Med* 82(1987):231–35.

Fell, J. C. "Drinking and Driving in America." *Alc Hlth Res Wd* 14(1990):18–25.

Fingarette, H. "Alcoholism: The Mythical Disease." In *Society, Culture, and Drinking Patterns Reexamined*, edited by D. J. Pittman and H. R. White. New Brunswick: Rutgers Center of Alcohol Studies, 1991.

Haller, E. "Eating Disorders: A Review and Update." *West J Med* 157(1992):658–62.

Hawley, D. A., et al. "Fatal Athletic Injuries." *Am J For Med Path* 8(1987):277–79.

Johnson, R. J. "Sudden Death during Exercise: A Cruel Turn of Events." *Post Med* 92(1992):195–206.

Keller, M., and J. Doria. "On Defining Alcoholism." *Alc Hlth Res Wd* 15(1991):253-259.

Klatsky, A. L., M. A. Armstrong, and H. Kipp. "Correlates of Liquor or Beer." *Br J Addic* 85(1990):1279–89.

Lehman, L. B., and S. J. Ravich. "Closed Head Injuries in Athletes." *Clin Sports Med* 9(1990):247–61.

Macewen, C. J. "Eye Injuries: A Prospective Study of 5671 Cases." *Br J Opht* 73(1989):888–94.

Mueller, F. O., and R. C. Cantu. "Catastrophic Injuries and Fatalities in High School and College Sports, Fall 1982—Spring 1988." *Med Sci Sports Exerc* 22(1990):737–41.

Perrine, M. W. B. "Who Are the Drinking Drivers? The Spectrum of Drinking Drivers Revisited." *Alc Hth Res Wd* 14(1990):26–35.

Pittman, D. J. "The New Temperance Movement." In *Society, Culture, and Drinking Patterns Reexamined*, edited by D. J. Pittman and H. R. White. New Brunswick: Rutgers Center of Alcohol Studies, 1991.

Roman, P. M. *Alcohol: The Development of Sociological Perspectives on Use and Abuse.* New Brunswick: Rutgers Center of Alcohol Studies, 1991.

Suh, I., et al. "Alcohol Use and Mortality from Coronary Heart Disease: The Role of High-density Lipoprotein Cholesterol." *Ann Intern Med* 116(1992):881–87.

Torg, J. S., and J. J. Vegso. "The National Football Head and Neck Injury Registry: 14-year Report on Cervical Quadriplegia (1971–1984)." *Clin Sports Med* 6(1987):61–72.

Vaillant, G. E. *The Natural History of Alcoholism.* Cambridge: Harvard Univ. Press, 1983.

Williamson, D. F., et al. "Smoking Cessation and Severity of Weight Gain in a National Cohort." *NEJM* 324(1991):739–45.

Wooley, S. C., and D. M. Garner. "Obesity Treatment: The High Cost of False Hope." *J Am Diet Assoc* 91(1991):1248–51.

Yager, J. "Has Our Healthy Life-style Generated Eating Disorders?" *West J Med* 157(1992):679–670.

CHAPTER 9: TEACH YOUR CHILDREN

American Council on Science and Health (ACSH). "The Responsible Use of Alcohol: Defining the Parameters of Moderation." *ACSH Newsletter,* 1991

Berg, L., and C. Homan. "Patterns of Consumption of Beer and Wine, Retail Availability and DUI." *J Alc and Drug Ed* (Dec. 1991).

DiNardo, J., and T. Lemieux. "Alcohol, Marijuana, and American Youth: The Unintended Effects of Government Regulation." *NBER Working Paper Series, no. 4212,* (Nov. 1992). Washington, D.C.: National Bureau of Economic Research.

Elias, M. "Kids' Aggression Linked to TV." *USA Today,* May 1993, sec. D1.

Engs, R. C. "Resurgence of a New 'Clean Living' Movement in the United States." *J School Health* 61[4](Apr. 1991):155–59.

Frost, D. "Crude Kids' TV Show Riles Marin Parents." *Marin Independent Journal,* July 1993.

Gelman, D. "The Violence in Our Heads." *Newsweek,* August 1993, 48.

Greenfield, M. "TV's True Violence." *Newsweek,* June 1993, 72.

Heath, D. B. "Beyond the Controversy: Education and Practical Sociocultural Alternatives." *Adol Coun* 9(Aug. 1989):3.

Jarvik, M. E. "The Drug Dilemma: Manipulating the Demand." *Science* 250(Oct. 1990):387–92.

Joseph, S. C. "Drug Policy in New York City." *Mt Sinai J Med (NY)* 58[5](Oct. 1991):421–22.

Koshland, D. E. "The New Puritanism." *Science* 248[4959](June 1990):1057.

———. "Scare of the Week." *Science* 244(1989):9.

KRT News Wire. "TV Violence Viewed as Public Health Threat to Kids." *Marin Independent Journal,* May 1993, sec. A, p. 17.

Mann, P. S. "Drugs and the Social Body." *Mt Sinai J Med (NY)* 58[5](Oct. 1991):427–32.

McCarthy, R. L., et al. "Product Information Presentation, User Behavior, and Safety." *Proc Human Factors Soc* 28(1984):81–85.

Millman, J., and F. Weldon. "Television Violence Under the Gun." *San Francisco Examiner*, June 1993, sec. D1.

Millman, R. B. "Pharmacology of the Drugs of Abuse and the Development of Public Policy." *Mt Sinai J Med (NY)* 58[5](Oct. 1991):416–20.

Rhodes, R. "Drug Use: Social and Scientific Background." Paper presented at the meeting of New York Regional Conference on Medical Ethics, New York, NY: March 1989. D.A. Moros, moderator.

Mulford, H. A., and J. L. Fitzgerald. "Consequences of Increasing Off-premise Wine Outlets in Iowa." *Br J Addic* 83(1988):1271–79.

Murtaugh, J. B. "Drug Use and Public Policy." *Mt Sinai J Med (NY)* 58[5](Oct. 1991):423–26.

National Institute on Alcohol Abuse and Alcoholism (NIAAA). *Seventh Special Report to the U.S. Congress on Alcohol and Health.* Rockville, MD: USDHHS, 1990.

Peele, S. "The Conflict between Public Health Goals and the Temperance Mentality." *Amer J Pub Health* 83(1993):6.

U.S. General Accounting Office. *Drug Abuse Prevention: Federal Efforts to Identify Exemplary Programs Need Stronger Design.* Gaithersburg, MD: GPO.

White, H., et al. "Learning to Drink: Familial, Peer, and Media Influences." In *Society, Culture, and Drinking Patterns Reexamined*, edited by D. J. Pittman and H. R. White. New Brunswick, NJ: Rutgers Center of Alcohol Studies, 1991.

World Health Organization (WHO). "Reducing Alcohol-related Problems." *Bull WHO* (1992):70(1).

Zeckhauser, R. J., and W. K. Viscusi. "Risk within Reason." *Science* 248(1990):559–63.

Zucker, R. A., and H. E. Fitzgerald. "Early Developmental Factors and Risk for Alcohol Problems." *Alc Health Res World* 15[1](1991): 18–24.

Index